Alzheimer's Disease: A Growing Concern

Alzheimer's Disease:
A Growing Concern

Edited by Blake Finn

hayle
medical

New York

Hayle Medical,
750 Third Avenue, 9th Floor,
New York, NY 10017, USA

Visit us on the World Wide Web at:
www.haylemedical.com

ISBN: 978-1-63241-742-8

Cataloging-in-Publication Data

Alzheimer's disease : a growing concern / edited by Blake Finn.
   p. cm.
Includes bibliographical references and index.
ISBN 978-1-63241-742-8
1. Alzheimer's disease. 2. Alzheimer's disease--Diagnosis. 3. Alzheimer's disease--Treatment.
4. Alzheimer's disease--Patients--Care. I. Finn, Blake.
RC523 .A49 2019
616.831--dc23

Table of Contents

Preface

Alzheimer's disease is a neurodegenerative disease which is considered to be the cause of most of the cases of dementia. It usually begins slowly and gradually worsens over time. Some of the main symptoms associated with Alzheimer's disease include difficulty in remembering recent events, problems with language, mood swings and disorientation. In severe cases, with a decline in condition, the patient's bodily functions are lost, ultimately leading to death. The cause of Alzheimer's disease in most of the cases is found to be genetic. Cognitive tests, blood tests and medical imaging are some of the common tests used to diagnose Alzheimer's disease. This book brings forth some of the most innovative concepts and elucidates the unexplored aspects of Alzheimer's disease. From theories to research, case studies related to all contemporary topics of relevance to this disease have been included herein. Coherent flow of topics, student-friendly language and extensive use of examples make this book an invaluable source of knowledge.

After months of intensive research and writing, this book is the end result of all who devoted their time and efforts in the initiation and progress of this book. It will surely be a source of reference in enhancing the required knowledge of the new developments in the area. During the course of developing this book, certain measures such as accuracy, authenticity and research focused analytical studies were given preference in order to produce a comprehensive book in the area of study.

This book would not have been possible without the efforts of the authors and the publisher. I extend my sincere thanks to them. Secondly, I express my gratitude to my family and well-wishers. And most importantly, I thank my students for constantly expressing their willingness and curiosity in enhancing their knowledge in the field, which encourages me to take up further research projects for the advancement of the area.

Editor

Gait Pathway in Subcortical Vascular Dementia and in Alzheimer's Disease

Rita Moretti, Arianna Sartori, Beatrice Baso and
Silvia Gazzin

Additional information is available at the end of the chapter

1. Introduction

Gait impairment, worse equilibrium scores and falls are associated with leukoaraiosis, as widely recognised [1-6]. In Binswanger's disease with a severe leukoaraiosis gait disorders are clearly evident while patients with mild periventricular changes may present subclinical forms of gait disorders, as proposed by some authors (see data in [7]).

Gait disorders in the elderly are particularly relevant, since they can influence the loss of functional independence and death [8]. As anticipated, cerebral small vessel disease (both white matter lesions and lacunar infarcts) correlates with gait parameters: stride length and a lower gait velocity [8]. Most importantly, subcortical vascular lesions seem to increase the possibility of falls, even if clear evidences are still lacking [9-11].

Walking difficulties in Alzheimer's disease are well described [12]: patients show slow and irregular steps, difficulties in turning and avoiding obstacles [13, 14]. These disturbances have been described also in patients free from extrapyramidal, ataxic, paretic signs, and clinically relevant musculoskeletal impairments [12, 14]. Moreover, Alzheimer's disease patients have a worse balance [12, 14, 15] and a higher risk of falls compared with matched controls [16, 17]. The prevalence of gait abnormalities varies widely across the studies (from 8.7% [18] to over 90% [19]); this can be explained because of different inclusion criteria and/or assessment procedures.

These observations have been confirmed by studies demonstrating that patients with Alzheimer's disease walk more slowly compared to healthy controls [12] and these gait problems have been interpreted as manifestations of the extrapyramidal deficits (well-known to affect

12–28% of Alzheimer patients), or as side effects of drug treatment (e.g. neuroleptic agents) [20]. Since a overt walking problems and trunk movement alterations can be seen also in absence of extrapyramidal signs, it has been proposed that some Alzheimer's disease patients may present "frontal gait disorder", a syndrome coterminous with gait apraxia [21, 15]. The lack of a standardised instrument to assess gait has been implicated as a possible cause for the low frequency of reports on the topic.

Since the walking assessment cannot discriminate between walking disorders caused by gait apraxia and other neurological causes of walking difficulty, there has been the necessity to exclude alternative causes of walking abnormalities in Alzheimer's disease (overt extrapyramidal impairments or other concurrent neurological diseases); in order to assess gait capacity, a new test has been proposed and a large proportion of the sample (40%) scored below cut off, even if the percentage of severely impaired was smaller. Although the possibility of right–left confusion, working memory deficits, and problems with verbal comprehension was minimised by demonstrating the items, the complexity of some of them might have contributed to inflating the proportion of patients performing poorly. Even though, the presence of associated vascular pathology in a few patients also cannot account for the outcome. Neuroradiological signs of white matter changes were reported in three of the 24 patients (22.5%) in the Della Sala *et al.*'s study [12], who scored below cut off in the assessment of walking skills.

Therefore, in a well-defined population suffering from subcortical vascular dementia and Alzheimer's disease (standing from a neurological, clinical, and radiological criteria), we tried to explore gait, balance and equilibrium alterations, and a behavioral complex symptom, such as apathy, even considering precipitant factors, such as concomitant pathologies and consequent therapies. We now present an extension of the work, with a speculation on what we observed for a two-year follow-up.

2. Subjects and methods

2.1. Patients

From June 1st 2010 to June 1st 2013, 155 patients diagnosed with Alzheimer's disease (AD), according to NINDCS-ADRDA criteria [22], and 673 patients with subcortical vascular dementia (according the NINDS-AIREN criteria for probable VaD [23]) (age 65–94 years) have been examined in Cognitive Disorder Unit Evaluation of the University of Trieste and enrolled in the present study.

The inclusion criteria were a Mini-Mental State Examination (MMSE) scores of at least 14 and satisfying the fourth edition of the Diagnostic and Statistical Manual of Mental Disorders (DSM-IV) criteria for dementia. As far as neuroimaging is concerned, subcortical VaD (sVAD) was diagnosed when the CT/MRI scan showed moderate to severe ischemic white matter changes [24] and at least one lacunar infarct. In order to be enrolled into the study, Alzheimer's subjects had to show on brain MRI the classical pattern of atrophy of AD (hippocampal atrophy) and display hypoperfusion in temporoparietal and precuneus regions (AD) on HMPAO-SPECT. The neurologist (RM) assessed independently, after the radiologist's opinion, brain CT and/or MRI images and all the diagnoses have been confirmed after a long term clinical follow-up (12 and 36 months).

Exclusion criteria were: normal pressure hydrocephalus, diagnoses of major stroke or brain haemorrhage, previous brain tumours, white matter lesions due to specific aetiologies (e.g. multiple sclerosis, vasculitis, brain irradiation, and genetic forms of vascular dementia such as CADASIL or CARASIL). Finally, also major psychiatric illness (e.g.. schizophrenia, bipolar disorders, psychosis, compulsive-obsessive disorders, etc) or central nervous system disorders and alcoholism were excluded. Also absence of an informed caregiver, unavailability of neuroradiological examination, and/or the use of psychotropic drugs within two months prior to the clinical assessment implied patient's exclusion from the study. According to these exclusion criteria, 27 AD patients and 70 sVAD patients were excluded. We did not consider a discriminant/exclusion criteria depression, referring to different studies (such as [25]), according to the potential correlation to vascular dementia predisposing factor.

2.2. Study design

This was a prospective cohort study, designed to investigate behavioural alterations, and in particular apathy of a AD and of a sVAD population. Study subjects underwent the following evaluations. The standardized baseline assessment implied a detailed history, physical examination (pulse rate and rhythm, blood pressure, heart size and sounds, peripheral pulses, retinal vessel and carotid artery evaluation), EKG, chest X-ray, laboratory tests and psychiatric evaluation. All patients were followed with neurological examinations scheduled every four months, while the complete neuropsychological examination was conducted at baseline and at 36 months. We conducted the study in accordance with the Declaration of Helsinki and with the Ethics Guidelines of the Institute.

2.3. Outcome measures

All patients were studied, with complete neurological and neuropsychological examinations. Main outcomes of the study were: global performance, which was assessed using the Mini Mental State Examination [26], Frontal Assessment Battery (FAB) [27]; global behavioral symptoms, assessed by the Neuro Psychiatric Inventory, NPI [28]; the caregiver stress, assessed by the Relative Stress Scale, RSS [29]. In addition to these main outcome measures, the Clinical Insight Rating Scale (CIR) [30] (which provides a measure of its four comprising items – awareness, cognitive deficit, disease progression and functional deficit) was performed. The Barthel index (BI) [31] and the Instrumental activity of Daily living (IADL) [32] have been used to assess functional activities and complex activities of daily living, respectively. Mobility problems were evaluated by the Tinetti scale for equilibrium/balance and gait [33]: in particular, a semiquantitative assessment was used, consisting of the modified Tinetti test with 17 items, 9 for body balance (0-16), 8 for gait (0-12). Patients were registered for their medical intake.

3. Statistical analysis

Statistical analyses were performed using the Statistical Package for the Social Sciences (SPSS, version 16.0). Wilcoxon Signed Ranks test was used to analyze the Within-group changes, from baseline to 24 months, of the overall scores for each efficacy variable.

Behavioral outcome measures, cognition, Tinetti scale, global, balance and equilibrium, and BI correlations were analyzed applying the Spearman's rank correlation analyses.

4. Results

The study subjects were 128 AD patients and 603 sVAD patients. All the patients could be fully studied (mean age 72.3 ± 7.3 years, range= 62-94 years). 1 AD patient and 5 sVAD patients died during the two-year follow-up. As anticipated, the diagnosis based on clinical history, neuropsychological assessment and neuroimaging was reinforced by subsequent follow-up in all cases.

All the selected patients underwent neuroimaging: 128 AD patients did MRI studies; 603 sVAD patients did CT scans; moreover, 201 of the latter completed the diagnostic pathway with MRI images, in case of not adequate imaging acquisition or not convincing data. Therefore, the patients who did CT/MRI were homogeneously recruited and no demographical/social/cultural/clinical difference distinguished from each other.

A neurologist (RM) revised all the imaging, employing the Blennow *et al.* [34] scale for CT scans and the Scheltens *et al.* [35] scale for MRI imaging in sVAD patients and Wahlund *et al.* [36], Kantarci *et al.* [37] and den Heijer *et al.* [38] criteria for AD MRI imaging. There was 95.8% inter-rater agreement for the independent assessment of the scans (kappa=0.8).

Patients were allowed to continue any previous therapy (e.g. antihypertensive, antidyslipidemic, antidiabetic drugs). During the follow-up, the patients were prescribed neuroleptics and/or benzodiazepines.

A synopsis of the cognitive performances obtained by the two groups has been reported in Table 1-2-3-4.

Baseline	sVAD	AD	P value (between groups)
MMSE	25.8 (2.4)	19.9 (1.9)	<0.01
Arithmetic calculations (WAIS) §	6.3 (1.6)	8.6 (1.2)	<0.05
Digit span forward (WAIS)	5.8 (1.5)	5.1 (0.6)	<0.05
Digit span backward (WAIS)	4.4 (2.5)	2.6 (0.8)	<0.05
FAB total score	9.2 (2.1)	11.8 (1.2)	<0.05

Table 1. Cognitive synoptical results obtained by the two groups studied. Values are mean (SD); ns = not significant. § number of mistakes.

24-month follow-up	sVAD within group (24 months vs baseline)	AD within group (24 months vs baseline)	P value (between groups)
MMSE	20.2 (2.2) (-5.2 (.0.3); p<0.01)	15.1 (1.7) (-4.85 (0.2); p<0.01)	<0.01
Arithmetic calculations (WAIS) §	5.4 (1.1) (-0.9 (0.5); ns)	3.4 (1.7) (-5.2 (0.5); p<0.01)	<0.05
Digit span forward (WAIS)	4.1 (1.4) (-1.7 (0.1); p<0.05)	3.2 (0.2) (-1.9 (0.4); p<0.05)	<0.05
Digit span backward (WAIS)	3.6 (0.3) (-0.8 (2.2); ns)	1.9 (0.1) (-0.5 (0.7); p<0.05)	<0.01
FAB total score	4.7 (1.5) (-4.5 (0.6); p<0.01)	7.5 (0.2) (-3.3 (1.0); p<0.05)	<0.01

Table 2. Cognitive synoptical results obtained by the two groups studied, at 12 months. Values are mean (SD); ns = not significant. § Number of mistakes. In brackets, in each column, comparison within group, 24 months *vs* baseline, reported as mean, SD, and p.

Tests	Baseline sVAD	Baseline AD
Barthel Index	87.41 ± 11.3	92.14 ± 0.11
Instrumental Activity of Daily Living	6.8 ± 0.34	5.84 ± 1.3

Table 3. TESTs results in the patients observed during follow-up.

Tests at 24 months	sVAD	AD	Between groups (sVAD vs AD)
Barthel Index	-25.17± 3.4 p<0.01	-13.57 ± 3.4 p<0.05	p<0.01
Instrumental Activity of Daily Living	-1.7 ± 0.3 p<0.05	-3.4 ± 3.4 p<0.01	p<0.01

Table 4. Results at 24 months: a comparison over baseline.

In summary, there are some important cognitive differences in the two groups: AD patients did worse in MMSE, in arithmetic calculation and in digit tasks of WAIS, IADL; sVAD patients did generally worse in FAB tests, Barthel Index.

From the behavioral perspective (Table 5-6), at baseline, the AD group had a worse score of NPI and BEHAVE-AD, and their caregivers did have a heavier stress (RSS). On the contrary, sVAD patients, at baseline did feel much more depressed (as stated by NPI partial scores, not purposely evaluated in this topic) and did have a better insight in their situation. After 24 months, AD patients showed higher NPI and Behave scores; sVAD patients did show more insight. Surprisingly, the stress levels of the caregivers were not significantly different in the two groups. sVAD patients did manifest more overt apathy, which increase during follow-up and remained a major key point in behavior disturbances of these patients.

Moreover, there was a dramatic decrease, either in gait and equilibrium control, either in the combined synoptical measure (of total score) in both groups, with sVAD patients showing a constantly worse performance, compared to AD patients (Table 7-8).

baseline	sVAD	AD	P value
RSS	24.7 (8.7)	36.1 (8.5)	(p<0.01)
NPI	16.9 (0.3)	24.4 (5.2)	(p<0.01)
CIR	3 (0.2)	2 (0.5)	(p<0.05)

Table 5. Behavioral synoptical results. Values are mean (SD); ns = not significant.

24-month follow-up	sVAD	AD	P value
RSS	47.5 (1.3) (+22.8 (5.9), <0.01)	45.2 (2.1) (+9.1 (6.8), <0.05)	ns
NPI	34.1 (0.8) (+17.2 (0.5), <0.01)	56.3 (4.5) (+31.9 (1.1), <0.01)	(p<0.01)
CIR	2.2 (0.3) (-0.8 (0.1), ns)	1.0 (0.3) (-1.0 (0.3), <0.05)	(p<0.01)

Table 6. Behavioral synoptical results. Values are mean (SD); ns = not significant; in brackets, in each column, comparison within group, 24 months *vs* baseline, reported as mean, SD, and p.

Tests	sVAD	AD	P value
TINETTI equilibrium	10.1 ± 0.1	14.3 ± 1.1	<0.001
TINETTI gait	10.2 ± 1.1	11.4 ± 0.3	<0.05
TINETTI tot. score	20.3 ± 1.2	25.7 ± 1.4	<0.001

Table 7. Gait TESTs results in the patients observed at baseline.

Tests at 24 months	Over baseline sVAD	Over baseline AD	Between groups (sVAD vs AD)
TINETTI equilibrium	-5 ± 0.6 p<0.01	-3.4 ± 0.6 p<0.01	P<0.001
TINETTI gait	-7.9 ± 1.1 p<0.01	-3.1± 1.1 p<0.01	P<0.001
TINETTI tot. score	-12.9 ± 0.2 p<0.01	-6.5 ± 0.2 p<0.01	P<0.001

Table 8. Results at 24 months: a comparison over baseline at 24 months.

Spearman's rank correlation analyses indicated that there was a significant correlation between Gait scores (total and separately, gait and equilibrium) and FAB scores (**total Tinetti score/ FAB**: r=0.81, *p* < 0.05 baseline; r=0.83, p < 0.01 over 24 months); **gait Tinetti score/FAB:** r=0.82, *p* < 0.01 over baseline; r=0.87, p < 0.01 over 24 months); **equilibrium Tinetti score/FAB:** r=0.81, *p* < 0.05 over baseline; r=0.83, p < 0.01 over 24 months) in sVAD.

Spearman's rank correlation analyses indicated that there was a significant correlation between Tinetti total, and equilibrium and gait score and BI over baseline, and 24 months (**total Tinetti score/BI**: r=0.81, *p* < 0.05 over baseline; r=0.89, p < 0.01 over 24 months); **gait Tinetti score/BI:** r=0.82, *p* < 0.01 over baseline; r=0.89, p < 0.01 over 24 months; **equilibrium Tinetti score/BI:** r=0.84, *p* < 0.01 over baseline; r=0.89, p < 0.01 over 24 months) in sVAD.

Furthermore, we have found a correlation between Tinetti equilibrium score and NPI over 24, months (equilibrium Tinetti/NPI: r=0.78, p<0.05 in sVAD; r=0.87, p<0.01 in AD), and Tinetti gait score and NPI over 24 months (**gait Tinetti /NPI**: r= 0.78, p<0.05 in sVAD; r=0.86, p<0.01 in AD), and Tinetti total score and NPI over 24 months (**Tinetti total score/NPI**: r= 0.78, p<0.05, in sVAD; r= 0.93, p<0.01 in AD).

Spearman's rank correlation analyses indicated that there was a significant correlation between Gait scores (total scores and separately, gait and equilibrium) and MMSE (**total Tinetti score/ MMSE**: r=0.81, *p* < 0.05 over 24 months in AD).

Surprisingly, we have found only a correlation between benzodiazepines intake and Tinetti equilibrium score at 24 months (respectively r=0.77, p<0.05 in sVAD; r=0.84, p<0.01 in AD).

We distinguished typical from atypical neuroleptic intake (Table 9). Moreover, since quetiapine, as an atypical neuroleptic, has a lower dopamine affinity compared to olanzapine, we considered separately the compounds, concluding as follows:

- Typical neuroleptics: a significant correlation between haloperidol intake and Tinetti equilibrium score at baseline and at 24 months (respectively: r=0.61, p<0.05, at baseline and r=0.81, p<0.01 in AD patients; r=0.72, p<0.05 at 24 months in sVAD); between haloperidol intake and Tinetti total score at baseline and 24 months (respectively: r=0.81, p<0.01 and r=0.86, p<0.01 in AD; only at 24 months r=0.71, p<0.01 in sVAD); not significant correlation between promazine chloridate intake and Tinetti sub-scores at baseline and at 24 months in AD; we have found a positive correlation between the equilibrium score of Tinetti test and promazine intake at 24 months in sVAD, not in AD group (r=0.74, p<0.05).

- Atypical neuroleptics: we have found a significant correlation between olanzapine intake and Tinetti equilibrium score at 24 months in AD groups (none of sVAD took olanzapine in our study) (r=0.74, p<0.05) and between olanzapine intake and Tinetti total score at 24 months (r=0.71, p<0.05); we have found a positive correlation between the equilibrium score of Tinetti test and quetiapine intake at 24 months (respectively: r=0.79, p<0.05 in AD group; r=0.82, p<0.01 in sVAD). The mean dose of olanzapine remained stable during the 24-month follow-up (5.2-5.4 mg/day); on the contrary, quetiapine dosage increased up to 24-month follow-up (56.3-89.6 mg/day).

Drug utilization	Baseline sVAD	24 months sVAD	Baseline AD	24 months sVAD
Benzodiazepines	144 patients	289 patients	298 patients	304 patients
lorazepam, mean (±SD) dose	1.27± 0.3 mg/day	2.56 ± 0.65 mg/day	3.94 ± 1.5 mg/day	4.56 ± 1.65 mg/day
delorazepam, mean (±SD) dose	1.21 ± 0.8 mg/day	2.61 ± 1.29 mg/day	3.1 ± 1.54 mg/day	4.1 ± 1.89 mg/day
bromazepam, mean (±SD) dose	2.11 ± 1.1 mg/day	3.41 ± 0.8 mg/day	4.6 ± 1.4 mg/day	5.41 ± 1.8 mg/day
Typical neuroleptics	88 patients	356 patients	88 patients	127 patients
haloperidol, mean (±SD) dose	1.56 ± 0.54 mg/day	2.34 ± 0.67 mg/day	2.87 ± 1.54 mg/day	3.56 ± 0.54 mg/day
promazine chloridrate, mean (±SD) dose	53.12 ± 12.23 mg/day	59.12 ± 16.91 mg/day	63.12 ± 7.2 mg/day	67.12 ± 1.56 mg/day
Atypical neuroleptics	4 patients	23 patients	63 patients	83 patients
olanzapine, mean (±SD) dose	0.0 ± 0 mg/day	0 ± 0 mg/day	5.6 ± 1.6 mg/day	5.9 ± 2.94 mg/day
quetiapine, mean (±SD) dose	37.5 ± 5.21 mg/day	56.9 ± 3.5 mg/day	66.8 ± 3.5 mg/day	89.9 ± 3.5 mg/day

Table 9. A synopsis of the CNS drugs employed by the patients.

5. Discussion

Walking is a complex mechanism, based on motor control, step rhythm, muscular activation and dys-activation, motor adjustment, attention, perception and so on. Spinal and brainstem activation, which seems to be fundamental for quadrupeds, is not so dominant in humans, where gait depends more on cortical and subcortical inputs [39].

The motor cortex, represented by distinct areas in the frontal lobes, receives a variety of inputs: sensory areas, motor control structures, and modulatory pathways including the thalamus and basal ganglia (BG). Movement planning and performance are strictly dependent from this cluster of architectonically distinct frontal fields [40]. In particular, SMA activates immediately before gait ignition in normal walking, suggesting a preparatory activity for each sub-component of a movement sequence [41]. It has been suggested that this activity may reflect sub-movement program selection, subsequently sent to the M1. On the other hand, BG generate a phasic activity, which switches off SMA output and which is probably involved in providing a non-specific cue both to trigger the sub-movement and to instruct the SMA to prepare for the next, finally generating an "automatic" movement sequence [42, 7]. In conclusion, internal cues give rise to automatic movement sequences, as a result of the cooperation of BG and SMA [7].

Gait control and in particular gait variability are deeply influenced by BG compensatory activity [43]. Rosano and colleagues reported that subclinical brain vascular abnormalities (WM infarcts and hyperintensities in MRI) were more frequent and severe in patients with a greater variability of step length, independently from age, gender, and cognitive function [43]. Moreover, older people and patients with leukoaraiosis show higher-level gait alterations, supporting the previous observations [39]. These data have been clinically confirmed by other works by the LADIS group [11], by Srikanth et al. [44] and by Masdeu and Wolfson [45].

Though, there are quite real differences among the few other studies on this point. It has been established by Della Sala *et al.* [12] that even AD, in a sizeable proportion (40% of their population) scored as having gait alteration. Though, it must be pointed out that the presence of associated vascular pathology, declared by the writers themselves is a not indifferent proportion (22.5%), even if they asserted that this could not account for the outcome. The Authors declared that their patients showed the gait apraxia phenomenon, referring to deficits of a relatively unitary function, with the reference to a theoretical model. Within the dichotomy, proposed by Benke [46], between a conceptual system of motor acts and a system which controls sensorimotor and spatial-temporal features of movement, gait apraxia would arise from the impairment of the latter system. Gait apraxia suggested Della Sala *et al.* [12] should also be distinguished from ideomotor apraxia, which hampers individual movements and meaningless gestures. What we observed in our study was the dramatically significant overcome of gait disturbances, either considering balance, either gait by itself, in pure sVAD rather than in pure AD pathology. Gait imbalance in AD relates with progressive and dramatic worsening of global cognitive functions (MMSE), with behavioural deterioration (NPI) and with consequent drugs intake.

On the contrary gait and balance in sVAD is a very precocious symptom, which relates, from the very beginning with frontal executive functions (FAB) and Barthel Index (BI) (Table 10).

Gait disturbances	sVAD	AD
	Peculiar	Unspecific
Characteristics	Early	Late
	Frequent	Less frequent
Relate to	Frontal executive functions (FAB)	Global cognitive functions (MMSE)
	Barthel Index (BI)	Behavioral performance (NPI)
		Drugs intake

Table 10. Summary: characteristics of gait disturbances in sVAD and AD patients.

Insofar, we hypothesize that even though gait apraxia is one of the symptoms declared in AD, affecting highly routinized synergistic actions, it relates to AD cognitive worsening. On the contrary, it is a key, precocious and very peculiar aspect of sVAD. Therefore, considering this point, it can be found a good explanation of the phenomenon, in Liston *et al.* [7] work; they suggested that microvascular alteration affecting the SMA, its connections in the periventricular WM, or the BG can cause a higher-level gait disorders (HLGDs), a hypothesis that seems to agree with the concept of gait apraxia caused by any mesial frontal lesion (SMA anatomical location) purposed by Meyer [47]. A further clinical confirmation is provided by current evidence of gait abnormities in early vascular dementia, in particular when WM alterations affect strategic pathways (linking the BG to the ventro-lateral nucleus of the thalamus and to the SMA and frontal areas) [48, 49]; these critical locations compromise the timing cues from the BG; the analogy to PD disconnections may suggest similar gait abnormalities. It is well known and widely accepted that leukoaraiosis is associated with gait impairment, falls, and worse equilibrium scores [1, 3-6, 8, 50]. Some authors suggest a spectrum of severity in gait disorders associated with WM abnormalities: on one side, severe gait disorder observed in Binswanger's disease with massive leukoaraiosis [7], on the other subclinical forms of gait disorders can occur in patients with mild periventricular changes.

However, it has been demonstrated that many patients with vascular-HLGDs present with disequilibrium as primary complaint rather than timing and movement ignition problems [4, 51, 7]. To explain this phenomenon it has been purposed that an alteration of the sensory/PMA pathways, compromising the contribute to sub-movements initiation and control of sensory input (proprioceptive, auditory, vestibular and visual information), may represent their primary disorder [7]. The preservation of BG/SMA pathways guarantees the generation of automatic, internally cued movements,

A clear point should be made in our study to the extremely strict exclusion criteria in AD and in sVAD recruitment, basically founded on clinical signs and neuroimaging world-wide accepted criteria. For example, in order to eliminate any confounding, we excluded patients with brainstem lesions, which ischemic lesions could cause specific gait and equilibrium abnormalities. Similarly, we considered also concurrent medications and co-morbidities, in order to ensure that the gait and balance alterations observed should be considered as an exclusive result of subcortical WM widespread damage. During the follow-up, a general worsening, decrease of behavioural control, and consequent pharmacologic intake (neuroleptics and benzodiazepines) stressed but did not cause directly the described gait abnormalities. In conclusion, it might be stated that subcortical lesions cause "per se" the interruption of long loop reflexes of deep white motor tracts and descending motor fibers arising from medial cortical areas (see data and literature in: Guerini *et al.* [10], Moretti *et al.* [52]), translating in gait alteration and imbalance. Moreover, subcortical vascular lesions involve fibres connecting frontal cortex and subcortical structures, which are responsible for motivation, executive function, planning and attention too (see in particular frontal eye fields). It has been suggested (see data and Literature in Moretti *et al.* [52]) that the basal ganglia maintains cortically selected motor set in the supplementary motor area and provides internal cues to the supplementary motor area in order to enable each sub movement to be correctly linked together [53-56].

Author details

Rita Moretti[1*], Arianna Sartori[2], Beatrice Baso[2] and Silvia Gazzin[3]

*Address all correspondence to: moretti@univ.trieste.it

1 Clinica Neurologica, Responsabile Ambulatorio Complicanze Internistiche Cerebrali, Dipartimento Universitario Clinico di Scienze Mediche, Chirurgiche e della Salute, Università degli Studi di Trieste, Italy

2 Clinica Neurologica, Dipartimento Universitario Clinico di Scienze Mediche, Chirurgiche e della Salute, Università degli Studi di Trieste, Italy

3 Area Science Park, FIF, Basovizza, Ospedale di Cattinara, Trieste, Italy

References

[1] Steingert A, Hachinski VC, Lau C, et al. Cognitive and neurologic findings in subjects with diffuse white matter lucencies on computed tomographic scan (leuko-araiosis). Arch Neurol. 1987;44(1):32–5.

[2] Junqué C, Pujol J, Vendrell P, et al. Leuko-araiosis on magnetic resonance imaging and speed of mental processing. Arch Neurol. 1990;47(2):151–6.

[3] Masdeu JC, Wolfson L, Lantos G, et al. Brain white matter changes in the elderly prone to falling. Arch Neurol. 1989;46 (12):1292–6.

[4] Baloh RW, Yue Q, Socotch TM, et al. White matter lesions and disequilibrium in older people. I. Case-control comparison. Arch Neurol. 1995;52(10):970–4.

[5] Mirsen TR, Lee DH, Wong CJ et al. Clinical correlates of white-matter changes on magnetic resonance imaging scans of the brain. Arch Neurol. 1991;48(10):1015–21.

[6] Inzitari D, Cadelo M, Marranci ML, et al. Vascular deaths in elderly neurological patients with leukoaraiosis. J Neurol Neurosurg Psychiatry 1997;62(2):177–81.

[7] Liston R, Mickelborough J, Bene J, et al. A new classification of higher level gait disorders in patients with cerebral multi-infarct states. Age Ageing. 2003;32(3):252–8.

[8] de Laat KF, van Norden AG, Gons RA, et al. Gait in elderly with cerebral small vessel disease. Stroke. 2010;41(8):1652-8.

[9] Guttmann CR, Benson R, Warfield SK, et al. White matter abnormalities in mobility impaired older persons. Neurology. 2000; 54(6):1277-83.

[10] Guerini F, Frisoni GB, Marrè A, et al. Subcortical vascular lesions predict falls at 12 months in elderly aptients discharged from a rehabilitation ward. Arch Phys Med Rehabil. 2008;89(8):1522-7.

[11] Baezner H, Blahak C, Poggesi A, et al. Association of gait and balance disorders with age-related white matter changes. Neurology. 2008;70(12):935-42.

[12] Della Sala S, Spinnler H, Venneri A. Walking difficulties in patients with Alzheimer's disease might originate from gait apraxia. J Neurol Neurosurg Psychiatry 2004;75(2): 196-201.

[13] Ala TA, Frey WH. Validation of the NINCDS-ADRDA criteria regarding gait in the clinical diagnosis of Alzheimer disease. A clinicopathologic study. Alzheimer Dis Assoc Disord. 1995;9(3):152–9.

[14] Alexander NB, Mollo JM, Giordani B, et al. Maintenance of balance, gait patterns, and obstacle clearance in Alzheimer's disease. Neurology. 1995;45(5):908–14.

[15] Visser H. Gait and balance in senile dementia of Alzheimer's type. Age Ageing. 1983;12(4):296–301.

[16] Buchner DM, Larson EB. Falls and fractures in patients with Alzheimer-type dementia. JAMA.1987;257(11):1492–5.

[17] van Dijk PT, Meulenberg OG, van de Sande HJ, et al. Falls in dementia patients. Gerontologist. 1993;33(2):200–4.

[18] Koller WC, Wilson RS, Glatt SL, et al. Motor signs are infrequent in dementia of the Alzheimer type. Ann Neurol. 1984;16(4):514–16.

[19] Fransenn EH, Kluger A, Torossian CL, et al. The neurologic syndrome of severe Alzheimer's disease. Relationship to functional decline. Arch Neurol 1993;50:1029–39.

[20] Burns A, Jacoby R, Levy R. Neurological signs in Alzheimer's disease. Age Ageing. 1991;20(1):45–51.

[21] Kurlan R, Richard IH, Papka M, et al. Movement disorders in Alzheimer's disease: More rigidity of definition is needed. Mov Disord 2000;15(1):24–9.

[22] McKhann G, Drachman D, Folstein M, et al. Clinical diagnosis of Alzheimer's disease: report of the NINCDS-ADRDA Work Group under the auspices of Department of Health and Human Services Task Force on Alzheimer's Disease. Neurology. 34(7): 939–44.

[23] Román GC, Tatemichi TK, Erkinjuntti T et al. Vascular dementia: diagnostic criteria for research studies. Report of the NINDS-AIREN International Workshop. Neurology. 1993;43(2):250- 60.

[24] Erkinjuntti T. Vascular dementia: challenge of clinical diagnosis. Int Psychogeriatr. 1997;9:77–83.

[25] Bus BA, Marijnissen RM, Holewjin S, et al. Depressive symptom clusters are differentialy associated with atherosclerotic disease. Psychol Med. 2011;41(7):1419-28.

[26] Folstein MF, Folstein SE, McHugh PR. "Mini-Mental state". A practical method for grading the cognitive state of patients for the clinician. J Psychiatr Res. 1975;12(3): 189–98.

[27] Dubois B, Slachevsky A, Litvan I, et al. The FAB: a Frontal Assessment Battery at bedside. Neurology. 2000;55(11):1621-6.

[28] Cummings JL, Mega M, Gray K, et al. The Neuropsychiatric Inventory: comprehensive assessment of psychopathology in dementia. Neurology. 1994;44(12):2308–14.

[29] Greene JG, Smith R, Gardiner M, et al. Measuring behavioural disturbance of elderly demented in patients in the community and its effects on relatives: a factor analytic study. Age Ageing. 1982;11(2):121–6.

[30] Ott BR, Lafleche G, Whelihan WM, et al. Impaired awareness of deficits in Alzheimer Disease. Alzheimer Dis Assoc Disord. 1996;10(2):68-76.

[31] Mahoney FI, Barthel DW. Functional evaluation: the Barthel Index. Md State Med J. 1965;14:61-65.

[32] Lawton MP, Brody EM. Assessment of older people: self-maintaining and instrumental activities of daily living. Gerontologist. 1969;9(3):179-86.

[33] Tinetti ME. Performance-oriented assessment of mobilty problems in elderly patients. J Am Ger Soc. 1986;34(2):119-26.

[34] Blennow K, Wallin A, Uhlemann C, et al. White-matter lesions on CT in Alzheimer patients: relation to clinical symptomatology and vascular factors. Acta Neurol Scand. 1991;83(3):187-93.

[35] Scheltens P, Barkhof F, Leys D, et al. A semiquantative rating scale for the assessment of signal hyperintensities on magnetic resonance imaging. J Neurol Sci. 1993;114(1): 7-12.

[36] Wahlund LO, Almkvist O, Blennow K, et al. Evidence-based evaluation of magnetic resonance imaging as a diagnostic tool in dementia workup. Top Magn Reson Imaging. 2005;16(6):427-37.

[37] Kantarci K, Jack CR Jr. Neuroimaging in Alzheimer disease: an evidence-based review. Neuroimaging Clin N Am. 2003;13(2):197-209.

[38] den Heijer T, Geerlings M, Hoebeek F, et al. Use of hippocampal and amygdalar volumes on MRI to predict dementia in cognitively intact elderly. Arch Gen Psychiatry 2006;63(1):57-62.

[39] Carboncini MC, Volterrani D, Bonfiglio L, et al. Higher level gait disorders in subcortical chronic vascular encephalopathy: a single photon emission computed tomography study. Age Ageing. 2009;38(3):302-7.

[40] Donoghue JP, Sanes JN. Motor areas of the motor cortex. J Clin Neurophysiol. 1994;11(4):382-96.

[41] Georgiou N, Iansek R, Bradshaw JL, et al. An evaluation of the role of internal cues in the pathogenesis of parkinsonian hypokinesia. Brain. 1993;116(Pt 6):1575–87.

[42] Phillips JG, Martin KE, Bradshaw JL, et al. Could bradykinesia in Parkinson's disease simply be overcompensation? J Neurol. 1994;241(7):439–47.

[43] Rosano C, Brach J, Studenski S, et al. Gait variability is associated with subclinical brain vascular abnormalities in high-functioning older adults. Neuroepidemiology. 2007;29(3-4):193-200.

[44] Srikanth V, Beare R, Blizzard L, et al. Cerebral white matter lesions, gait and risk of incident falls: a prospective population based study. Stroke. 2009;40(1):175-80.

[45] Masdeu JC, Wolfson L. White matter lesions predispose to falls in older people. Stroke. 2009;40(9):e546.

[46] Benke T. Two forms of apraxia in Alzheimer's disease. Cortex. 1993; 29(4):715-29.

[47] Meyer JS, Barron DW. Apraxia of gait: a clinico-physiological study. Brain.1960;83(2): 261–84.

[48] Hennerici MG, Oster M, Cohen S, et al. Are gait disturbances and white matter degeneration early indicators of vascular dementia? Dementia. 1994;5(3-4):197–202.

[49] Moretti R, Torre P, Antonello RM, et al. The on-freezing phenomenon: cognitive and behavioural aspects. Parkinsons Dis. 2011; Article id:746303;1-7.

[50] Junque C, Pujol J, Vendrell P et al. Leuko-araiosis on magnetic resonance imaging and speed of mental processing. Arch Neurol. 1990;47(2):151–6.

[51] Waite LM, Broe GA, Creasey H, et al. Neurological signs, aging, and the neurodegenerative syndromes. Arch Neurol. 1996;53(6):498–502.

[52] Moretti R, Torre P, Antonello RMA. Basal ganglia: functional and organic roles in behavior and cognition. Nova Science Publishers Inc, New York; 2009.

[53] Iansek R, Bradshaw JL, Phillips JG, et al. Interaction of the basal ganglia and supplementary motor area in the elaboration of movement. In: Glencross DJ, Piek JP (ed.) Motor control and sensorimotor integration. Amsterdam: Elsevier Science; 1995. p37–59.

[54] Lee AC, Harris JP. Problems with perception of space in Parkinson's disease: a questionnaire study. Neuro-Ophthalmology 1999;22(1):1-15.

[55] Almeida QJ, Frank JS, Roy EA, et al. An evaluation of sensorimotor integration during locomotion toward a target in Parkinson's disease. Neuroscience. 2005;134(1): 283-93.

[56] Gurvich C, Georgiou-Karistianis N, Fitzgerald PB, et al. Inhibitory control and spatial working memory in Parkinson's disease. Mov Disord 2007;22(10):1444-50.

2

Uncontrolled Sexual Behaviour in Dementia

Susan van Hooren and Wim Waterink

Additional information is available at the end of the chapter

1. Introduction

Uncontrolled sexual behaviour in dementia is considered as a symptom of the behavioural disturbances seen in dementia, such as agitation, disinhibition, apathy, depression, and psychotic behaviour. The combination of these behavioural problems and progressive cognitive dysfunctions are the main characteristics of dementia. The behavioural problems, are present in 80-95% of the patients with dementia [1]. These symptoms decrease the quality of life of patients, increase the likelihood of institutionalization, and contribute most to caregivers burden. Although less common than most other behavioural problems, uncontrolled sexual behaviour is often more disruptive and upsetting to a spouse, institutional staff and other residents [2-4]. Therefore, these sexual behaviours are a tremendous challenge for health care providers in institutional care settings. However, a literature search utilizing Pubmed showed that only 0,5% of the literature addressing dementia concerns sexual functioning, and even less focuses on uncontrolled sexual behaviour. Thus, uncontrolled sexual behaviour is a serious neglected area in this field, while the majority of health care providers agree that more information and institutional training is needed [2, 5, 6].

2. Uncontrolled sexual behaviour

Uncontrolled sexual behaviour is labelled and defined in many ways in the literature. Synonyms used are 'Disinhibited sexual behaviour' [7], 'Inappropriate sexual behaviour' [8, 9], 'Inappropriate sexual expression' [2], 'Increased sexual activity' [10], and 'Hypersexuality' [11]. All phrases imply that this behaviour is a sexual act (verbal or physical) which is unacceptable, inappropriate, disinhibited, or uncontrolled within the (social) context in which it is carried out. Examples are sexual comments, masturbation in public, grabbing at the genitals and/or breasts of other persons, chasing other residents for sexual purposes, and exposing one's genitals in public. Some of these behaviours may be inappropriate only because they are performed in public and therefore should not be confused with sexual appetite and behaviour in older people due to a normal sex drive. There is no widely agreed definition of when this behaviour becomes inappropriate and so it is subject to subjective interpretation of the observer. In this chapter, 'uncontrolled' is used reflecting a reduced capacity to manage an impulsive response to a situation.

There are several types of behaviours identified in the literature to cluster uncontrolled sexual behaviour. In some reviews of the literature, three types were suggested, i.e. sex talk, sexual acts, and implied sexual acts [11-13]. Sex talk is regarded as the most common form and involves inappropriate language, that is not in line with the patient's premorbid personality. Sexual acts include touching grabbing, exposing or masturbating in public or in private settings. Implied sexual acts involve reading pornographic material in public or requesting unnecessary genital care. In an observational study that included 40 patients with dementia living in a nursing home [14], research assistants scored whether exposed sexual behaviour was appropriate, ambiguous or inappropriate. The patients were systematically observed on nine separate five minute occasions in the nursing home during different situations, such as at meals, being groomed or dressed, in their rooms. Most sexual behaviour was coded as inappropriate or ambiguous. Overall, this scoring leaves substantial gaps for individual interpretation of the observer. Besides, the three types of sexual behaviour were not based on empirical evidence.

More recently, two observational studies shed more light on the definition and measurement of uncontrolled sexual behaviour. In the first study [15], sexual behaviours were observed and afterwards clustered in several types. Based on an observational study which included 12 patients with dementia, aged between 53 and 84 years of age, nineteen sexual behaviours were obtained from observations and interviews with their caregivers and categorised by the authors in three types, i.e. 'sexual acts with contact with others', 'sexual acts with non-contact with others', and 'verbal sexual behaviour'. The most frequently observed sexual behaviours consisted of patients stroking their own genitals in private, touching areas of another person and verbal provocation. In the second study [16], 68 health professionals were questioned, working in institutions with patients with progressive neurological disease or patients with acquired brain injury, which resulted in 145 examples of uncontrolled sexual behaviours. Incidents of touching others inappropriately was the most common uncontrolled sexual behaviour.

Based on the abovementioned study in which an observation instrument was developed [16, 17], items were identified for the development of a questionnaire regarding sexual behaviour in dementia (SBDQ; [6]). The questionnaire consisted of four discrete behaviour categories: verbal comments, non-contact behaviour, exposure, and touching others. 115 health professionals were asked to rank the behavioural descriptors in terms of severity. This resulted in four levels of severity for each behaviour category. The rankings resulted in categorisations of uncontrolled sexual behaviours that are more evidence based and initiated a methodological tool that may have value for clinical use and research purposes. The validity and reliability of this scale was investigated and established (see also, [6]).

3. Uncontrolled sexual behaviour in dementia

Because of the limited coverage of uncontrolled sexual behaviour within the literature and the use of different definitions and categorisations, it is difficult to obtain a robust view of prevalence of these behaviours in dementia. Nevertheless, there are some studies which offer an insight in the frequency of uncontrolled sexual behaviour in dementia. For example, Burns et al. (1990) found that 7% of 178 patients with Alzheimer's disease showed sexual inappropriate behaviour (i.e. exposure, obscene sex language, masturbation, propositioning others). A more recent study [19] showed nearly a similar prevalence rate (8%) of references to sexual behaviour in medical records of 165 older people with dementia living in a residential care facility. The prevalence is substantially lower in a mixed cohort with patient living in nursing homes and patients living in the community. Of the 2278 participants only 41 (i.e. 1,8%) had a documentation of verbal or physical aberrant sexual behaviour [8]. In an observational study, there was a clear difference in prevalence rates between types of dementia, such as Alzheimer's disease, vascular dementia, pick's disease [14]. Patients with Alzheimer's disease expressed less uncontrolled sexual behaviour compared to patients diagnosed with other types of dementia (i.e. 9% versus 28%). This difference was also seen in other studies. For example, Alagiakrishnan (2005) demonstrated that 53,6% of the patients expressing uncontrolled sexual behaviour were diagnosed with vascular dementia, while 22% was diagnosed with Alzheimer. And even in the sample of twenty patients expressing uncontrolled sexual behaviour of De Medeiros et al. (2008), this difference was significant (p<0.01). The higher percentages of uncontrolled sexual behaviour in non-Alzheimer's types of dementia may be explained by a relatively higher likelihood of brain pathology that is associated with hyper sexuality (e.g. striatum, frontal lobes, temporo-limbic system and hypothalamus (e.g. [12]).

It not clear whether uncontrolled sexual behaviour is more prevalent in men than women or in patient with more severe dementia. Most studies only included men and dementia severity was often not investigated with regard to uncontrolled sexual behaviour. In studies that focused on uncontrolled sexual behaviour and included severity of dementia, the results were inconclusive. Burns et al. (1990) found a positive association with severity of dementia, while De Medeiros et al. (2008] concluded that half of the subjects with uncontrolled sexual behaviour had mild dementia, whereas most subjects with non-sexual behaviours had severe dementia. However, this difference did not reached significance. In both studies the frequency of sexual behaviour was equal for men and women, while two other studies have shown that sexual behaviour was more prevalent in men [5, 8].

In sum, based on these cross-sectional studies, prevalence rates of uncontrolled sexual behaviour in dementia vary between 1,8%-28%, which depends on type of dementia.

4. Etiology

The etiology of uncontrolled sexual behaviour is rather complex and must be considered within a biopsychosocial perspective [20]. Generally, the literature attributes this behaviour to biological changes associated with dementia, such as changes in brain structures and/or neurotransmitters. Case studies demonstrated that dysfunction of interconnected brain structures may cause uncontrolled sexual behaviour. Four major brain systems have been suggested [12, 13], i.e. the frontal lobes, the temporo-limbic system, the striatum, and the hypothalamus. Head trauma to the frontal and temporal lobes may decrease inhibitory impulses often needed to keep sexual feeling in control and therefore result in uncontrolled sexual behaviour. Pick's disease and Kluver-Bucy syndrome is associated with frontal and temporal pathology. These patients are characterized by social inappropriate behaviour, including uncontrolled sexual behaviour. Injury to the striatal region, as in Huntingtons and Parkinson disease, may result in obsessive-compulsive sexual behaviour [21]. Lesions to the right hypothalamus can cause manic symptoms, including increased sexual desire.

Psychological factors may also contribute to uncontrolled sexual behaviour or maintain this behaviour. First, some behavioural problems, including depression, hyperactivity, or mania, may increase sexual interest and result in uncontrolled sexual behaviour [19]. Other diagnoses, such as delirium, epileptic seizures and alcohol abuse may also cause uncontrolled sexual behaviour [7, 21]. Second, the amount of sexual interest is also determined by premorbid patterns of sexual activity [20]. Third, uncontrolled sexual behaviour may be due to disorientation, which is often seen in the patient with dementia. For example, because of the cognitive impairments, the patient with dementia may not be aware of his or her surroundings, and display behaviour considered normal in private but not in public. Similarly, a patient may misidentify another person as their spouse, and display behaviour appropriate for a married couple [9].

Psychosocial factors that may be associated with uncontrolled sexual behaviour are lack of a usual partner, lack of privacy, or an under stimulating environments. Older adults in residents may lack physical closeness, especially when they don't have a partner. Physical closeness might reduce loneliness and anxiety of the patient with dementia. When this need is not met, it is possible that this may take the form of physical aggression in persons not knowing how to appropriately meet their needs for closeness and intimacy. In nursing homes, there is often a lack of privacy and less opportunities for patients to be intimate with their partner. This may even be aggravated by the relatively passive and conservative attitude in some health professionals toward older people sex issues [2, 5]. In addition, an under stimulating environment may increase boredom and loneliness, which may result in disruptive sexual behaviour. In conclusion, the etiology of uncontrolled sexual behaviour is rather complex and there are many factors that could cause or maintain uncontrolled sexual behaviour.

Empirical studies addressing the etiological factors of uncontrolled sexual behaviour in dementia are very sparse. Since uncontrolled sexual behaviour may have an immense impact on patients and their relationship with others, family, caregivers, and institutional staff, it is important to gain more information on uncontrolled sexual behaviour and its etiology. More insight in uncontrolled sexual behaviour in dementia and the etiology, would be useful in diagnosing symptoms of uncontrolled sexual behaviour and could provide directions for interventions in order to help the patient, health professionals, and families to deal with this behaviour.

5. Management

The management of uncontrolled sexual behaviour is often a challenge. Less is known about the best way to act, while the need for evidence based guidelines is growing. Overall, management of uncontrolled sexual behaviour can be divided in behavioural strategies and

pharmacological treatment. Because many of the drugs carry significant risk of adverse side effects, it is important to start with a solid assessment of the situation (including the degree of risk to others) and appropriate behavioural treatment.

5.1. Assessment

First of all, the exact target behaviour, context and involved factors need to be defined; what form? In what context? Frequency? What factors contribute? What is known from the (sexual) history? Is it a desire for closeness, comfort, or lack of privacy? Is it a problem and to whom? Are there any risks and to whom? Do the patient have insight? What is the mental/cognitive status? [12, 20]. These questions may be answered by direct observation of the patient, in an open discussion with main staff and significant others, and/or a standardised measurement, like the SBDQ [6]. In addition, it is important to rule out delirium and consider mood disorders or psychosis. These disorders need other management than uncontrolled sexual behaviour. Examining physical status and current medications is needed to determine (bio)medical causes. Different classes of medications have shown to induce uncontrolled sexual behaviour, in clinical settings [22]. For example, atypical antipsychotics can induce uncontrolled sexual behaviour by blocking the effects of selective serotonin reuptake inhibitors [23]. The reason for this is, that selective serotonin reuptake inhibitors typically suppresses sexual drive [7, 24-26]. In sum, a careful assessment provides information to choose an appropriate treatment (strategy) and a good baseline to properly evaluate the process and the effects of treatments.

5.2. Behavioural treatment

After a careful assessment, it is possible to develop a care plan with the involved care professionals and it is recommended to involve significant others. A care plan may include elements that are directed to the patient, significant others, other residents, and the staff. To the patient, many behavioural strategies may be initiated depending on the form of behaviour, the contributing factors, and the patients cognitive functioning (possibilities for new learning). Examples of behavioural strategies are distraction during presence of uncontrolled sexual behaviour via substitution of other activities, redirecting via conversation or humour, ignore unwanted behaviour and encourage appropriate behaviour, modification of social cues that are being misinterpreted, removing 'triggers' of the behaviour, substitute caregivers to the sex that does not match their sexual preference, avoidance of external cues such as over stimulating television or radio programs, trousers that open in the back or with zippers in case of exposing behaviour, providing single rooms, "not disturb" signs, and/or allowing doors to remain shut to provide privacy to let the patient satisfy their sexual needs [9, 12, 27-29]. To the significant others or spouses it is useful to give additional information to reframe the behaviour and reassurance that these behaviours are not a reflection of their relationship.

Providing staff supervision and additional education may be extremely helpful, because care professionals report that it is often difficult to cope with these behaviours or it is distressing for them [2, 30]. There should be a good balance between openness to the patients need for normal sexual expression while preventing uncontrolled sexual behaviour [12]. It is also critical to prepare students for uncontrolled sexual behaviour. In a study in which a young student introduced herself to several residents, she was confronted with uncontrolled sexual behaviour and responded with guilt, confusion, and distress [30]. More reflection on own behaviour and small changes in the appearance, like another manner of dressing, may help in provoking less uncontrolled sexual behaviour. In addition, providing more information on the etiology of the behaviour may aid to reduce guilt and confusion of the student or care professional. Because students and care professionals may be uncomfortable discussing uncontrolled sexual behaviour, it is important that the supervisor initiates the topic and provide coping strategies to them. Specific methods, like role playing, may be quite helpful to prepare the student for uncontrolled sexual behaviour [30].

After all, it is important that evidence based guidelines will be developed in addition to a policy and procedures within an organisation.

5.3. Pharmacological treatment

Different classes of medication (e.g. antidepressant, antiandrogen, antipsychotic, and anticonvulsant medications) have been proposed in the treatment of uncontrolled sexual behaviour [31]. The basis for medication treatment comes from the similarities of paraphilias with sexual behaviour [32]. Paraphilias and hypersexual behaviour, both involve uncontrolled sexual behaviour. Hence, pharmacological treatment of uncontrolled sexual behaviour is focused on pharmacological agents that affect monoamine neurotransmitters and that enhance central serotonergic function in particular (see also, [33]). However, there is not yet convincing data supporting the use of a particular medication. Most evidence is in the form of case reports and data are also lacking with regard to the advantage of any medication over placebo or in comparison with other medications [31, 34].

Author details

Susan van Hooren[1,2*] and Wim Waterink[1]

*Address all correspondence to: Susan.vanhooren@ou.nl or susan.vanhooren@zuyd.nl

1 Faculty of Psychology and Educational Sciences, Open University of the Netherlands, The Netherlands

2 Zuyd University of Applied Sciences, Heerlen, The Netherlands

References

[1] Aalten P, De Vugt ME, Jaspers N, Jolles J, Verhey FR. The course of neuropsychiatric symptoms in dementia. Part II: relationships among behavioural sub-syndromes and the influence of clinical variables. Int J Geriatr Psychiatry. 2005;20(6):531-6.

[2] Holmes D, Reingold J, Teresi J. Sexual expression and dementia. Views of caregivers: A pilot study. Int J Geriatr Psychiatry. 1997;12(7):695-701.

[3] Mayers KS. Sexuality and the patient with dementia. Sexuality and disability. 1994;12(3):213-9.

[4] Mayers KS, McBride DC. Sexualized components of verbally abusive statements by residents with dementia diagnoses. Sexuality and disability. 1996;14(2):109-16.

[5] Archibald C. Sexuality, dementia and residential care: managers report and response. Health Soc Care Community. 1998;6(2):95-101.

[6] Bartelet M, Waterink W, Van Hooren S. Extreme sexual behavior in dementia as a specific manifestation of disinhibition. Journal of Alzheimer's Disease. 2014;42:S119-S24.

[7] Alkhalil C, Tanvir F, Alkhalil B, Lowenthal DT. Treatment of Sexual Disinhibition in Dementia: Case Reports and Review of the Literature. American Journal of Therapeutics. 2004;11(3):231-5.

[8] Alagiakrishnan K, Lim D, Brahim A, Wong A, Wood A, Senthilselvan A, et al.. Sexually inappropriate behaviour in demented elderly people. Postgrad Med J. 2005;81(957):463-6.

[9] Kamel HK, Hajjar RR. Sexuality in the nursing home, part 2: Managing abnormal behavior-legal and ethical issues. J Am Med Dir Assoc. 2003;4(4):203-6.

[10] Haussermann P, Goecker D, Beier K, Schroeder S. Low-dose cyproterone acetate treatment of sexual acting out in men with dementia. Int Psychogeriatr. 2003;15(2): 181-6.

[11] Wallace M, Safer M. Hypersexuality among cognitively impaired older adults. Geriatr Nurs. 2009;30(4):230-7.

[12] Black B, Muralee S, Tampi RR. Inappropriate Sexual Behaviors in Dementia. Journal of Geriatric Psychiatry and Neurology. 2005;18(3):155-62.

[13] Ozkan B, Wilkins K, Muralee S, Tampi RR. Pharmacotherapy for inappropriate sexual behaviors in dementia: a systematic review of literature. Am J Alzheimers Dis Other Demen. 2008;23(4):344-54.

[14] Zeiss AM, Davies HD, Tinklenberg JR. An observational study of sexual behavior in demented male patients. Journal of Gerontology. 1996;51:M325-M9.

[15] Tzeng Y, Lin L, Shyr YL, Wen J. Sexual behaviour of institutionalised residents with dementia – a qualitative study. J Clin Nurs. 2009;18(7):991-1001.

[16] Knight C, Alderman N, Johnson C, Green S, Birkett-Swan L, Yorstan G. The St Andrew's Sexual Behaviour Assessment (SASBA): development of a standardised recording instrument for the measurement and assessment of challenging sexual behaviour in people with progressive and acquired neurological impairment. Neuropsychol Rehabil. 2008;18(2):129-59.

[17] Johnson C, Knight C, Alderman N. Challenges associated with the definition and assessment of inappropriate sexual behaviour amongst individuals with an acquired neurological impairment. Brain Injury. 2006;20(7):687-93.

[18] Burns A, Jacoby R, Levy R. Psychiatric phenomena in Alzheimer's disease. IV: Disorders of behaviour. British Journal of Psychiatry. 1990;157:86-94.

[19] De Medeiros K, Rosenberg PB, Baker AS, Onyike CU. Improper sexual behaviors in elders with dementia living in residential care. Dement Geriatr Cogn Disord. 2008;26(4):370-7.

[20] Series H, Degano P. Hypersexuality in dementia. Advances in psyciatric treatment. 2005;11:424-31.

[21] Guay DR. Inappropriate sexual behaviors in cognitively impaired older individuals. Am J Geriatr Pharmacother. 2008;6(5):269-88.

[22] Bardell A, Laus T, Fedoroff JP. Inappropriate sexual behaviour in a geriatric population. International Psychogeriatrics. 2011;23(7):1182-8.

[23] Lam MHB, Fong SYY, Wing Y-K. Sexual disinhibition in schizophrenia possible induces by risperidone an quetiapine. Psychiatry and Clinical Neuroscience. 2007;61(333).

[24] Baldwin DS. Sexual dysfunction associated with antidepressant drugs. Exp Opin Drug Safety. 2004;4/3:457-70.

[25] Jacobsen FM. Fluoxetine-induced sexual dysfunction and an open trial of yolimbine. Journal of Clinical Psychiatry. 1992;53:119-22.

[26] Levinsky AM, Owen NJ. Pharmacological treatment of sexual inhibition in dementia. Case reports and review of the literature. American Journal of Geriatric Soc 1999;47:231-4.

[27] Lesser JM, Hughes SV, Jemelka JR, Griffith J. Sexually inappropriate behaviors. Assessment necessitates careful edical and psychological evaluation and sensitivity. Geriatrics. 2005;60(1):34-7.

[28] Buhr GT, White HK. Difficult behaviors in long-term care patients with dementia. J Am Med Dir Assoc. 2006;7:180-92.

[29] Tsatali MS, Tsolaki MN, Christodoulou TP, Papaliagkas VT. The Complex Nature of Inappropriate Sexual Behaviors in Patients with Dementia: Can We Put it into a Frame? Sexuality and disability. 2011;29(2):143-56.

[30] Mayers KS. Inappropriate social and sexual responses to a female student by male patients with dementia and organic brain disorder. Sexuality and disability. 2000;18(2):143-7.

[31] Joller P, Gupta N, Seitz DP, 'Frank C, Gibson M, Gill SS. Approach to inappropriate sexual behaviour in people with dementia. Can Fam Physician. 2013;59(3):255-60.

[32] Krueger RB, Kaplan MS. The paraphilic and hypersexual disorders. An overview. Journal of Psychiatric Practice. 2001;7(391-403).

[33] Kafka MP. The monoamine hypothesis of the pathophysiology of paraphilic disorders: An update. In: Prentky RA, Janus ES, Seto MC, editors. Sexually coercive behaviour Understanding and management. New York: New York Academy of Sciences.; 2003. p. 86-94.

[34] Mania I, Evcimen H, Mathews M. Citalopram Treatment for Inappropriate Sexual Behavior in a Cognitively Impaired Patient. Prim Care Companion J Clin Psychiatry. 2006;8(2):106.

3

Free Cholesterol — A Double-Edge Sword in Alzheimer Disease

José C. Fernández-Checa

Additional information is available at the end of the chapter

1. Introduction

Alzheimer's disease (AD) is a progressive neurodegenerative disorder that accounts for most of dementia cases in elder people. The main features of AD include a progressive deterioration of intellectual functions, most prominently memory impairment, loss of language ability, and cognitive deficits. Motor defects appear in the late phases of the disease and basic activities of daily living are gradually compromised as the pathology progresses to advanced phases, and are often accompanied by psychosis and agitation [1, 2]. The hallmarks of the disease include the accumulation of amyloid-β peptide (Aβ) inside neurons and in the extracellular brain space, and the intracellular formation of neurofibrillary tangles (NFTs) composed of hyper-phosphorylated tau protein, loss of synapses at specific brain sites as well as the degeneration of cholinergic neurons from the basal forebrain [3]. The prevalence of AD is about 8–10 % of the population over 65 years of age, which increases 2-fold every 5 years afterwards [4, 5]. This high rate prevalence together with the increase in life expectancy, point to AD as one of the most serious health concerns wordlwide, whose incidence is expected to tiple in the next 2-3 decades unless more effective therapies are available [6].

The identification of new targets for the development of more effective therapeutic approaches requires a better understanding of the molecular pathways leading to AD. In this regard, both genetic and environmental factors are increasingly recognized to contribute to the development of AD, which occurs in two forms. The sporadic form of the disease, which affects people over 65 years of age and accounts for the vast mayority of AD cases. In a small proportion (6–8 %), the disease is inherited as an autosomal dominant trait and appears as an early onset in people younger than 65 years of age. Mutations within three genes, the amyloid precursor protein (APP) gene on chromosome 21, the presenilin 1 (PSEN1) gene on chromosome 14, and the presenilin 2 (PSEN2) gene on chromosome 1, have been identified as the main cause of early onset familial AD [7-10]. While these findings are key for our understanding of the pathogenesis of familial AD, these mutations account for 30–50% of all autosomal dominant early onset cases.

In the last years, it has become increasingly recognized that cholesterol plays a significant role in AD. The first evidence of the importance of cholesterol was the discovery that the ε4 allele of the cholesterol transport protein apolipoprotein E (ApoE) is associated with a higher risk of developing both familial and sporadic AD and modulates the age of AD onset [11-14]. Despite these findings, the impact and causal role of cholesterol in AD remains controversial (see below), as exemplified by the inconsistent outcome of statins in modulating AD risk and progression, which calls for the need for large-scale trials to document whether statins and cholesterol modification regulate or modify the course of AD [15, 16]. Emerging data, however, position the small pool of cholesterol in mitochondria as a key player in AD by determining the susceptibility of neurons to Aβ neuroinflammation, synaptotoxicity and neurotoxicity and as a culprit of cognitive decline by depleting specific mitochondrial antioxidant defense mechanisms. In this review, we will briefly summarize the role of cholesterol in AD, focusing not only in the evidence that cholesterol may foster the amiloidogenic processing of APP and the generation of Aβ peptide, but most importantly, recent findings indicate that cholesterol trafficking to mitochondria stands as a novel critical factor that sensitizes to Aβ-induced neuroinflammation and neurotoxicity, emerging as a potential target for intervention.

2. The involvement of Aβ and cholesterol in AD

2.1. The role of Aβ in AD

Since Aβ was first identified as a component of amyloid plaques, increasing evidence has suggested that Aβ is a major player in AD pathogenesis. According to the amyloid cascade hypothesis, the dysregulation of APP metabolism and Aβ deposition are primary events in the onset of the disease [17, 18]. The Aβ 1–42 and Aβ 1–40 peptides are the major forms found in amyloid plaques, which are generated by proteolytic cleavage of APP. These plaques are predominantly found in areas affected by neurodegeneration, such as entorhinal cortex, amygdala, neocortex, and particularly, hippocampus [19, 20]. While the number of plaques usually does not correlate with the severity of dementia, clinical correlation between elevated Aβ deposition in the brain and cognitive decline has been reported [21]. As described below, several lines of evidence suggest that overproduction and/or reduced clearance of Aβ peptides are key to amyloid aggregation, which contributes to the development of NFTs and neurodegeneration in AD pathology. Intraneuronal Aβ can derive by either APP cleavage within neuronal endocytic compartments, as well as by Aβ internalization from the extracellular space. Both sources are of relevance in the formation of the pool of Aβ involved in neurodegeneration. Intraneuronal Aβ accumulation is one of the earliest pathological events in humans and in animal models of AD, which correlates with early abnormalities in long term potentiation (LTP), cognitive dysfunctions and precedes the formation of amyloid plaques and NFTs formation and the neurodegeneration in animal models in which intracellular Aβ and neuronal loss have been reported [22-26]. Furthermore, Aβ plaques could generate from the death of neurons that contained elevated amounts of Aβ and this release can account for the loss of intraneuronal Aβ immunoreactivity in areas of plaque formation [24, 27, 28]. Moreover, recent findings indicated that internalized Aβ elicits fibrillization in the multivesicular bodies (MVBs), which after reaching the plasma membrane, cause cell death and the release of amyloid structures into the extracellular space, indicating that exosomes derived from MVBs could release part of the intracellular pool of Aβ to contribute to the extracellular Aβ pool [29, 30]. The contribution of intracellular Aβ to neuronal death has been well documented in cortical neurons from brains of AD and Down syndrome patients that undergo apoptosis after accumulation of Aβ42 [31, 32]. In addition, microinjection of Aβ1-42 or cDNA-expressing cytosolic Aβ1-42 induces cell death in primary human neurons, while neuronal loss associated with intracellular accumulation of Aβ has been described in a transgenic APP(SL)PS1KI mouse that closely mimics the development of AD-related neuropathological features of AD [33, 34]. Intracellular Aβ accumulation has been associated with neuritic and synaptic pathology and transgenic mice harboring constructs that target Aβ intracellularly developed neurodegeneration [35-37]. Furthermore, antibodies against Aβ reduced intraneuronal Aβ accumulation prevented synaptotoxicity and reversed cognitive impairment in triple transgenic mice [22, 38]. Finally, a coding mutation (A673TT) in APP has been recently shown to protect against AD and age-related cognitive decline in elderly Icelanders [39]. This mutation that affects the aspartyl protease β-site in APP significantly reduces the formation of amyloidogenic peptides, strongly indicating that reducing the β-cleavage of APP protect against the disease. Thus, although targeting Aβ may be a rationale approach to prevent or treat AD progression, recent findings have unfolded the diversity of Aβ structures revealed by the immune response to fibrillar Aβ [40]. This outcome may account for the failure of single therapeutic monoclonal antibodies against Aβ in the treatment of AD.

2.2. Amiloidogenic processing of APP and Aβ generation

Amiloidogenic processing of APP yields toxic Aβ peptides (Fig 1). In this pathway, the β- and γ-secretases cleave APP at the N- and C-termini of the Aβ peptide, respectively. APP, β - secretase, PS1 and Aβ are all present in lipid rafts, which are enriched in cholesterol and glycosphingolipids. This led to the suggestion that APP in lipid rafts is primarily processed via the β-secretase, and APP outside of ratfs is processed via the α-secretase pathway. β-secretase has been characterized as a membrane-bound aspartic protease termed beta-site APP-cleaving enzyme 1 (BACE1), while γ-secretase is a complex comprised of presenilin-1 or -2, nicastrin, anterior pharynx-defective 1 (Aph-1) and presenilin enhancer 2 (Pen-2) [41]. β-arrestin 2, is a novel member of the γ-secretase complex that physically associates with the Aph-1α subunit of the γ-secretase complex and redistributes the complex toward detergent-resistant membranes, increasing the catalytic activity of the complex [42]. Moreover, β-arrestin 2 expression is elevated in individuals with AD and its overexpression leads to an increase in Aβ peptide generation, whereas genetic silencing of Arrb2 (encoding β-arrestin 2) reduces generation of Aβ in cell cultures and in Arrb2-/- mice. In addition to its amyloidogenic processing by β- and γ-secretases, APP can be cleaved within the Aβ domain by α-secretase. This non-amyloidogenic processing prevents the deposition of intact Aβ peptide and results in the release of a large soluble ectodomain, sAPPα, from the cell, which has neuroprotective and memory-enhancing effects. Members of the ADAMs, a disintegrin and metalloprotease family of proteases, have been shown to possess α-secretase activity [43].

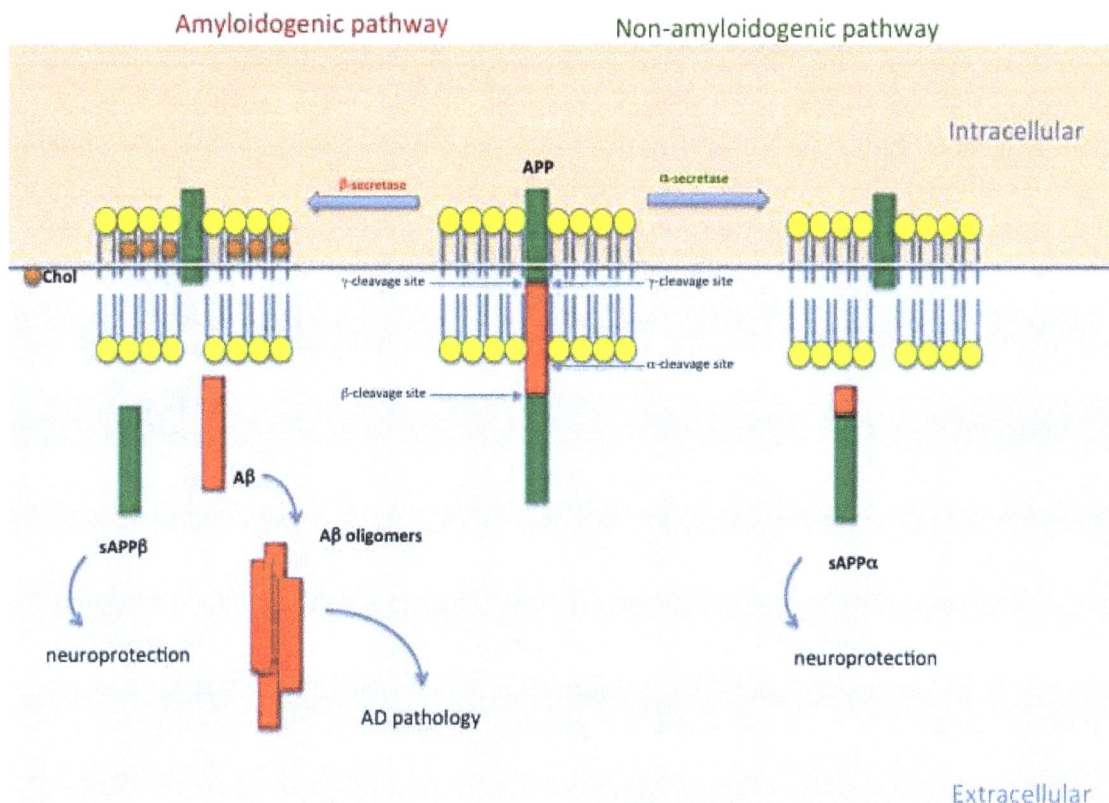

Figure 1. Role of membrane cholesterol in amyloidogenesis. β- and γ-secretases cleave APP at the N- and C-termini of the Aβ peptide, respectively. APP, β-secretase, PS1 and Aβ are all present in lipid rafts, which are enriched in cholesterol and glycosphingolipids. Therefore, APP in lipid rafts is primarily processed via the β-secretase, and APP outside of ratfs is processed via the α-secretase pathway. In the former, β-secretase-mediated Aβ peptides oligomerize and accumulate in plaques contributing to the neurotoxicity of AD.

Besides its extracellular deposition, current evidence indicates the processing and targeting of APP and Aβ to intracellular sites, including mitochondria [44]. Moreover, levels of mitochondrial APP are higher in affected brain areas and in subjects with advanced disease symptons [45]. Immunoelectron microscopy analyses indicated the association of APP with mitochondrial protein translocation components, TOM40 and TIM23, which correlated with decreased import of respiratory chain subunits *in vitro*, decreased cytochrome oxidase activity, increased ROS generation and impaired mitochondrial reducing capacity [45].

2.3. The role of cholesterol in AD: facts and controversies

Cholesterol is an essential component of membrane bilayers that regulate structral and functional properties and, hence, a pleiotropic number of cell functions and in the intracellular trafficking of proteins [46]. Cholesterol is required for synapse formation, biogenesis of synaptic vesicles and regulation of neurotransmitter release and the precursor of steroid hormones and oxysterols, which are critical intermediates in many metabolic pathways [47-49]. Cholesterol homeostasis is altered in AD; however, whether cholesterol levels are upregulated or downregulated in AD remains to be established. The pathogenic processing of APP into toxic Aβ fragments is known to occur in cholesterol-enriched membrane domains of the plasma membrane, called lipid rafts. The first evidence that cholesterol may impact Aβ production in the brain came from observations that dietary cholesterol increases amyloid production in rabbit hippocampal neurons [50]. Work in mice genetically modified to deposit cerebral Aβ demonstrated that a cholesterol-enriched diet resulted in increased Aβ deposition and increased amyloid plaque formation [51], and these observations were confirmed in subsequent studies in mice fed diets enriched in cholesterol [52-55]. As discussed below, very little cholesterol is transferred from the periphery to the brain due to the impermeability of the blood brain barrier (BBB), so the observations of diet-induced cholesterol-mediated Aβ deposition in neurons are puzzling. A potential explanation for these findings is the fact that BBB permeability is impaired in AD [56, 57]. Exploiting the relative detergent insolubility of lipid rafts, there has been evidence indicating the localization of APP, the α-, β- and γ-secretases in rafts [58, 59]. In addition, the activities of BACE1 and γ-secretase are stimulated by lipid components of rafts, in particular glycosphingolipids and cholesterol. Consistent with these findings supporting a role for cholesterol in AD pathogenesis, high cholesterol levels have been shown to correlate with Aβ deposition and the risk of developing AD [60-62]. Patients taking the cholesterol-lowering drug statins have a lower incidence of the disease [62, 63]. Besides ApoE, other genes encoding proteins involved in cholesterol homeostasis, including cholesteol 24-hydroxylase (CYP46A1), the acyl-coenzyme A:cholesterol acyltransferase (ACAT), the cholesterol efflux transporters ABCA1 and ABCA7, and the lipopotrein-receptor-related protein (LRP) have been linked to the risk, development or progression of AD [64-68]. Despite this experimental and epidemiological evidence, the role of increased cholesterol in AD is controversial with findings showing the opposite. For instance, earlier studies indicated that hippocampal membranes of AD brains showed a reduced fluidity in the hydrocarbon core region compared to control subjects that correlated with the cholesterol content in AD samples [69]. Moreover, reduced cholesterol levels and cholesterol/phospholipids mole ratio have been reported in the temporal gyrus but unaffected in the cerebellum of AD patients with respect to controls [70]. Decreased 24-hydroxycholesterol levels that correlated with lower lathosterol content was reported in the frontal and occipital cortex of patients with AD compared to subjects controls [71]. In addition, cholesterol levels were slightly increased in frontal cortex gray matter in AD patients with the ApoE4 genotype compared with ApoE4 control subjects [72]. Finally, neuronal membrane cholesterol loss has been shown to enhance Aβ generation in hippocampal membranes from AD patients exhibiting increased colocalization of BACE1 and APP [73], and hippocampal membranes from the brain of AD patients contain less membrane cholesterol than control [74]. Furthermore, it has been reported that inhibition of the mevalonate pathway increased production of Aβ and amyloid plaques [75]. Prospective cohort studies have failed to demonstrate the protective effect of statins on dementia, while others reports did not replicate the Aβ lowering effect of statins in the cerebrospinal fluid [76-81]. In addition to these findings arguing against the correlation between increased brain cholesterol and AD, there is evidence that both cholesterol and Aβ reciprocally regulate each other and that Aβ impacts negatively in cholesterol synthesis, in part, by inhibiting stero-regulated element binding proteins-2 (SREBP-2) cleavage [82, 83]. Interestingly, the consequent decrease in protein prenylation contributes to Aβ-induced neuronal death, which is reversed by exogenous supply of isoprenoids. Further work is needed to ascertain whether the intracellular distribution rather than the levels of brain cholesterol levels may correlate with disease severity.

3. Regulation of cholesterol metabolism in the brain

3.1. De novo cholesterol synthesis

Compared with other organs, the brain is the highest cholesterol-containing organ, which is present mainly in unsterified form. Most of the free cholesterol pool is localized predominantly in specialized membranes (myelin) and to a lesser extent in neurons and glial cells. Experimental evidence indicates that brain cholesterol is independent of serum cholesterol levels, as the BBB is impermeable to circulating cholesterol, which determines that both neurons and glial cells synthesize cholesterol *de novo*. Oligodendrocytes control the synthesis of myelin and therefore have the highest capacity to synthesize cholesterol, followed by astrocytes [84, 85]. Cholesterol is synthesized from acetate in a multistep cascade that requires oxygen and energy. The precursor acetyl-CoA is first converted to 3-hydroxy-3-methylglutaryl-CoA (HMG-CoA) and then to mevalonate (Fig. 2). The phosphorylation of mevalonate yields 5-pyrophospho-mevalonate, which is converted to isopentenyl pyrophosphate (IPP). IPP can be reversibly transformed to dimethylallyl pyrophosphate (DMAPP), and the combination of both IPP and DMAPP yields the 10-carbon isoprenoid geranyl pyrophosphate (GPP). The sequential addition of 1 or 2 more IPP units to GPP generates the 15-carbon and the 20-carbon isoprenoids farnesyl pyrophosphate (FPP) and the geranylgeranyl pyrophosphate (GGPP), respectively. FPP branches into the non-sterol pathways, which contributes to the generation of other derivatives such as ubiquinol, dolichol, and the sterol pathway via conversion into squalene by squalene synthase, which catalyzes the first committed step in cholesterol synthesis. The rate-limiting step of cholesterol biosynthesis is the conversion of HMG-CoA to mevalonate catalyzed by the HMG-CoA reductase (HMGCR), which is bound to endoplasmic reticulum (ER). Cholesterol levels control HMGCR through several mechanisms. First, high cholesterol exerts a feedback inhibition by activating HMGCR ubiquitination and subsequent proteasomal degradation. Moreover, HMGCR expression is regulated by ER-bound transcription factor SREBP-2, which in turn is controlled by a sterol-sensitive SREBP cleavage-activating protein (SCAP) [86]. In the presence of sterols, full-length SREBP-2 is restricted to the ER. Upon sterol depletion, SREBP-2 interacts with SCAP and is transported from the ER to the Golgi apparatus, where SREBP-2 is cleaved by two proteases and the released N terminus domain acts as a transcription factor to subsequently enhance the levels of HMGCR [86, 87]. Thus, ER plays a key role in the supply of endogenous cholesterol synthesis, which operates to meet demand for cell cholesterol.

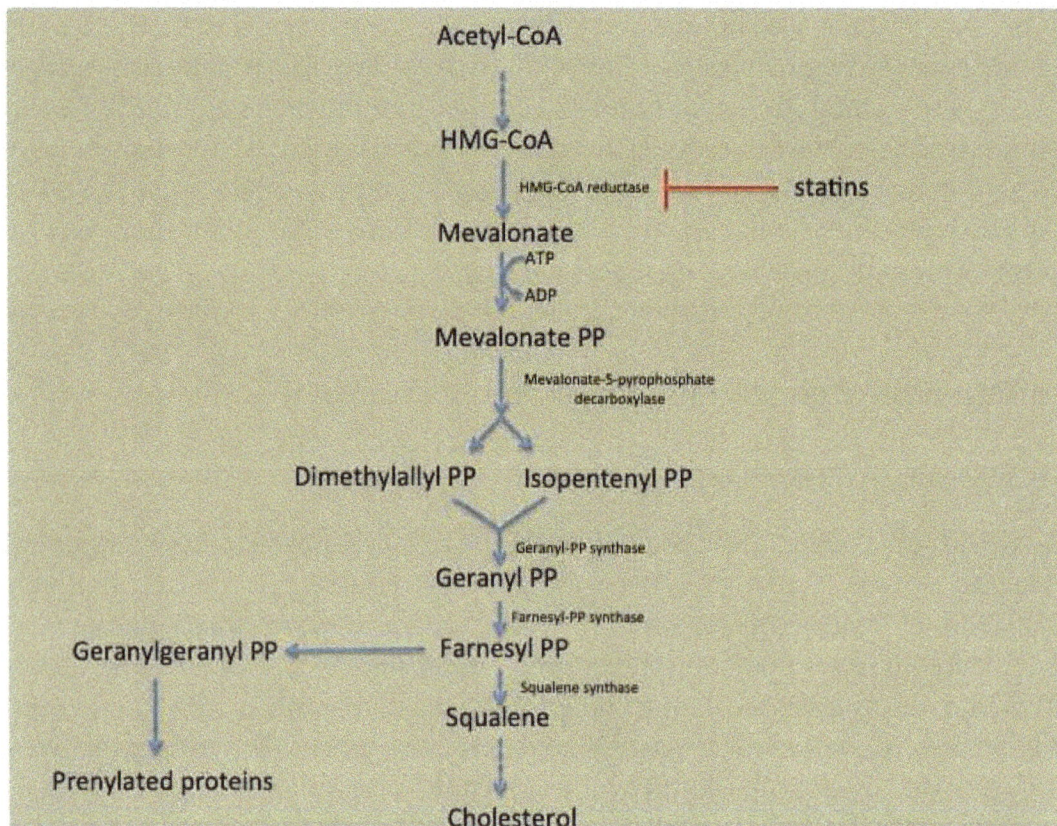

Figure 2. Cholesterol synthesis in the mevalonate pathway. Cholesterol is synthesized from acetate in a multistep cascade that requires oxygen and energy. The precursor acetyl-CoA is first converted to 3-hydroxy-3-methylglutaryl-CoA (HMG-CoA) and then to mevalonate. This pathway also generates isoprenoids. Farnesyl pyrophosphate (FPP) branches into the non-sterol pathways, which contributes to the generation of other derivatives such as ubiquinol, dolichol, and the sterol pathway via conversion into squalene by squalene synthase, which catalyzes the first committed step in cholesterol synthesis. The rate-limiting step of cholesterol biosynthesis is the conversion of HMG-CoA to mevalonate catalyzed by the HMG-CoA reductase (HMGCR), which is the target of statins. Statins hence will not only block cholesterol synthesis but also isoprenoids and other non-sterols, which may account for the pleiotropic effects of statins.

3.2. Cholesterol storage and transport

In contrast to developing neurons, which synthesize most of the cholesterol required for growth and synaptogenesis, mature neurons depend on the availability of exogenous cholesterol derived from astrocytes (Figure 3). This process not only ensures steady supply of cholesterol to neurons but also spares energy, as ATP hydrolysis is required to synthesize cholesterol de novo [88]. Besides de novo synthesis, astrocytes can also internalize and recycle the cholesterol released from degenerating nerve terminals and deliver it back to neurons [89]. The transport of cholesterol from astrocytes to neurons requires binding to one of the variants of ApoE, the most prevalent lipoprotein in the central nervous system. In this process, cholesterol first forms a complex with ApoE, which is then secreted in a process involving ABCA1 and ABCG1 transporters [90, 91]. Using cultured cerebellar murine astroglia cells, it has been shown that partially lipidated apoE, secreted directly by glia, is likely to be the major extracellular acceptor of cholesterol released from glia in a process mediated by ABCG1 rather than ABCA1 [91]. The secreted ApoE–cholesterol complex is then internalized into neurons predominantly via the LDL receptor (LDLR) as well as LRP, and to a minor extent by very-low-density lipoprotein receptor (VLDL), ApoE receptor 2, and megalin [92]. The specific contribution of these receptors in the uptake of ApoE-cholesterol complex and hence in the maintenance of neuronal cholesterol homeostasis remains to be established. Once internalized the receptor-bound ApoE–cholesterol complex is delivered to the late endosomes/lysosomes where acid lipase hydrolyses the cholesterol esters within the lipoprotein complex, resulting in the release of intracellular free cholesterol. This unesterified cholesterol subsequently exits the late endosomes/lysosomes via Niemann–Pick type C (NPC) 1 and 2 protein-dependent mechanism and is distributed primarily to the plasma membrane as well as to the ER, which serves as a negative feedback sensor for the cholesterol homeostasis genes such as HMGCR and LDLR. Excess cholesterol, on the other hand, is esterified in the ER by ACAT and stored in cytoplasmic lipid droplets, which serves as reserve source of cholesterol needed for synaptic and dendritic formation and remodeling [93, 94].

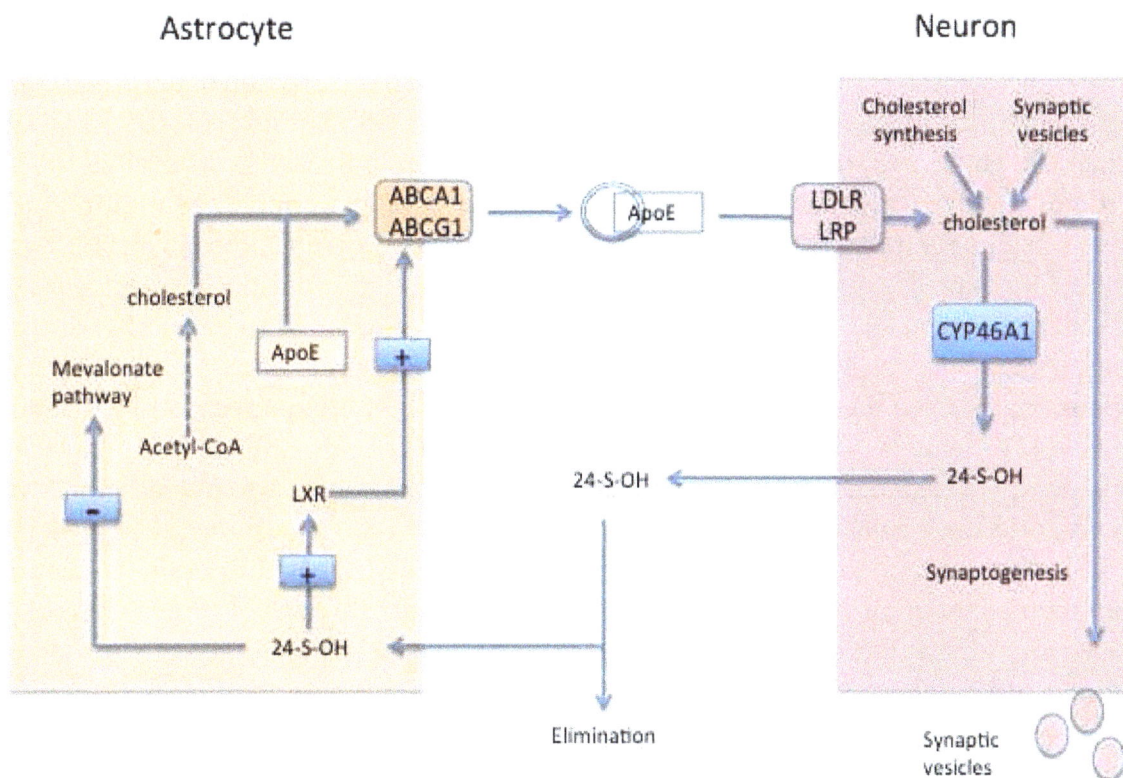

Figure 3. Cross talk between astrocytes and neurons in cholesterol homeostasis. Although neurons can synthesize cholesterol de novo in the adult state neurons rely on the delivery of cholesterol from astrocytes, which exhibit a significantly higher rate of de novo cholesterol activity than neurons. Cholesterol packed in ApoE particles assembled in astrocytes are delivered via ABCA1 carrier to neurons. Excess neuronal cholesterol is transformed into the oxysterol 24S-hydroxysterol (24S-OH) by the CYP46A1 which represents the major mechanism for the elimination of brain cholesterol, as it crosses the BBB to the periphery for disposal. Oxysterols activate transcription factor LXRβ isoform, which in turn induces the activation of carriers such as ABCA1 to stimulate trafficking of cholesterol in the form of ApoE to neurons. 24S-OH inhibits the novo cholesterol synthesis in astrocytes.

3.3. Cholesterol efflux from the brain

Unlike other organs and epithelial cells, neurons and glial cells do not degrade cholesterol, therefore in order to maintain homeostasis they export cholesterol to the circulation for its disposal by peripheral organs. Two different mechanisms are involved in the elimination of cholesterol from the brain. The major mechanism by which cholesterol is excreted from the brain is by its conversion to 24S-hydroxylcholesterol—an oxidized lipophilic metabolite that can freely cross the BBB [95]. The conversion of free cholesterol to 24S-hydroxycholesterol is mediated by the cytochrome P450-containing enzyme cholesterol 24-hydroxylase, encoded by the Cyp46A1 gene, which is expressed selectively in the brain [96]. High levels of this enzyme are found in certain neuronal cells such as pyramidal neurons of the hippocampus and cortex, Purkinje cells of the cerebellum, thalamic neurons, and in hippocampal and cerebellar interneurons. Interestingly, a minor fraction of cholesterol 24-hydroxylase immunoreactivity has also been detected in glial cells from the brains of AD patients [95]. It is estimated that about 40% of the total cholesterol turnover is mediated by cholesterol 24-hydroxylase [97]. Indeed, deletion of the Cyp46A1 gene encoding cholesterol 24-hydroxylase leads to about 50% reduction in brain cholesterol excretion. This decrease, however, is compensated by the reduction in de novo synthesis, thus suggesting a close relationship between synthesis and metabolism of cholesterol in the brain. The other mechanism of cholesterol elimination, called reverse cholesterol transport pathway, involves translocation of a fraction of brain cholesterol to the blood by membrane transport protein such as ABCA1 [98]. The level of ABCA1 is partly regulated by cholesterol-derived ligand oxysterols (e.g., 24S-hydroxylcholesterol) of the liver X receptor (LXR), which has been shown to influence the transcription of multiple genes involved in cholesterol metabolism [99-101]. There are two known LXR isoforms, LXRα and LHRβ. LXRα expression is mainly limited to the liver, adrenals, intestine and spleen, while LXRβ is expressed in all tissue types, including the brain. In vivo induction of LXR results in increased expression of ABCA1 and ABCG1, increased cholesterol efflux and a reduction in synaptosomal plasma membrane cholesterol [101]. As such, it is expected that LXR agonists (e.g. T0901317) should lower Aβ levels. However, results with LXR agonists have been inconsistent. For instance, T0901317 has been shown in some studies to decrease Aβ, while others reported an increase in Aβ42 without chaning Aβ40 levels [102]. Hence, it is conceivable that both synthesis and elimination of cholesterol, especially in the adult brain, are not only tightly regulated but also compartmentalized. Astrocytes are responsible for the majority of cholesterol synthesis but contribute relatively little to its elimination, whereas neurons with reduced synthetic ability can eliminate about two thirds of the cholesterol from the brain.

4. Intracellular cholesterol and AD

As a key component of membrane bilayers, intracellular cholesterol traffics to different compartments to maintain physical and functional membrane properties. Cholesterol that enters the cell via the endocytic pathway is transported to the ER for processing, while cholesterol synthesized in the ER de novo it is transported to the plasma membrane within a short time frame. Of relevance to AD pathogenesis, in the following sections we will focus on the endo-lysosomal cholesterol and in the small pool of cholesterol in mitochondria and their contribution to AD.

4.1. Endo-lysosomal cholesterol

The supply of cholesterol from astrocytes to neurons via receptor-bound ApoE-cholesterol complex relies on the trafficking and subsequent hydrolysis of these complexes in endo/ lysosomes. The generated free cholesterol exits lysosomes via NPC1/2 proteins to be distributed to other membrane bilayers. The impact of NPC proteins in intracelular cholesterol homeostasis has been best characterized in the NPC disease, a neurological disorders caused by mutations in NPC1/2 proteins characterized by increased accumulation of cholesterol and other lipids (e.g. glycosphingolipids) in lysosomes in the affected organs, predominantly brain and liver. NPC knockout mice, which mimic the pathology of NPC patients, exhibit increased lysosomal cholesterol in cerebellum, mainly in Purkinje cells, and suffer from progressive motor deterioration and a short life span (typically 8-10 weeks). NPC disease and AD share many parallels including endo/lysosomal abnormalities and APP processing and Aβ accumulation. Previous findings have shown that mutated NPC1 in mice causes the accumulation of Aβ40 and Aβ42, which coincided with accumulation of presenilins in early endocytic compartment [103]. Similar findings have been reported in human NPC1 brain, with accumulation of Aβ ocurring in early endosomes [104]. In CHO cells deficient in NPC1 protein and in cells treated with U18666A, which inhibits NPC1/2, Aβ and presenilin accumulation were found in late endosomes [105]. However, the expression of NPC1 in AD has been poorly characterized. Quite intriguingly, recent findings have reported increased expression of the lysosomal cholesterol transporter NPC1 in AD [106]. NPC1 expression was described to be upregulated at both mRNA and protein levels in the hippocampus and frontal cortex of AD patients compared to controls subjects. However, no difference in NPC1 expression was detected in the cerebellum, a brain region that is relatively spared in AD. Moreover, murine NPC1 mRNA levels increased in the hippocampus of 12-month-old APP/PS1 mice compared to wild type mice. While these findings strongly suggest the lack of lysosomal cholesterol accumulation in AD, endosomal abnormalities have been found in AD that precede amyloid and tau pathology in the neocortex. In addition to the proteolytic processing by secretases, APP and its corresponding C-terminal fragments are also metabolized by lysosomal proteases. SORLA/SORL1 is a unique neuronal sorting receptor for APP that has been causally implicated in sporadic and autosomal dominant familial AD. Brain concentrations of SORLA are inversely correlated with Aβ in mouse models and AD patients. Indeed, transgenic mice overexpressing SORLA exhibit decreased Aβ concentrations in brain [107]. Mechanistically, Aβ binds to the amino-terminal VP10P domain of SORLA and this binding is impaired by a familial AD mutation in SORL1. Although previous studies have shown that lysosomal cholesterol accumulation impairs autophagy by disrupting lysosomal function [108], the lysosomal impairment and subsequent contribution to decreased Aβ degradation in AD may occur through mechanisms independent of cholesterol accumulation in lysosomes. Moreover, sphingosine-1-phosphate (S1P) accumulation by S1P lyase deficiency has recently been shown to impair lysosomal APP metabolism, resulting in increased Aβ accumulation [109]. The intracellular accumulation of S1P interferes with the maturation of cathepsin D and degradation of Lamp2, suggesting a general impairment of lysosomal function and autophagy. Sphingolipids have strong affinity to bind cholesterol and play a role in Alzheimer disease [110]. However, it remains to be established whether increased lysosomal cholesterol may contribute to impaired lysosomal Aβ degradation and if sphingolipids accumulate in lysosomes in AD.

4.2. Mitochondrial cholesterol

Unlike plasma membrane, mitochondria are cholesterol-poor organelles. The limited pool of mitochondrial cholesterol plays important physiological roles, such as in the synthesis of steroids in specialized tissues and bile acids in the liver. However, under pathological conditions the unphysiological accumulation of cholesterol in mitochondrial membranes have profound effects in mitochondrial function and antioxidant defense and has emerged as an important factor in liver diseases and neurodegeneration [111-114]. In particular, the transport of cholesterol from the outer to the inner mitochondria is essential for the generation of steroid precursor pregnenolone upon metabolism of cholesterol by the P540 side-chain cleavage enzyme CYP11A1. Availability of cholesterol in mitochondria inner membrane is rate-limiting step in steroidogenesis and is a highly regulated process.

StARD1 is the founding member of a family of lipid transporting proteins that contain StAR-related lipid transfer (START) domains. StARD1 is an outer mitochondrial membrane protein which was first described and best characterized in steroidogenic cells where it plays an essential role in cholesterol transfer to the mitochondrial inner membrane for metabolism by CYP11A1 to generate pregnenolone. Despite similar features with StARD1, other START members cannot replace StARD1 deficiency as global StARD1 knockout mice dye within 10 days due to adrenocortical lipoid hyperplasia [115]. These findings imply that other members of the family cannot functionally replace StARD1, indicating the key role of this member in the regulation of cholesterol trafficking to the mitochondrial inner membrane. Recent findings in APP/PS1 models of AD have indicated the expression of StARD1 in neurons, which correlate with the age-dependent increase in mitochondrial cholesterol [114, 116]. Consistent with these findings in experimental models, enhanced immunocytochemical localization of StARD1 has been described in the pyramidal hippocampal neurons of AD-affected patients [117]. Given the role of StARD1 in the mitochondrial transport of cholesterol and hence in the modulation of mitochondrial cholesterol levels, the increased expression of StARD1 in AD patients, would strongly suggest that mitochondrial cholesterol accumulation may actually occur in patients with AD. Furthermore, the increase in mitochondrial cholesterol in brain mitochondria of Alzheimer's disease was not accompanied by a selective increase in mitochondrial-associated membranes (MAM), a specific membrane domain made of ER and mitochondria bilayers thought to be of relevance in the traffic of lipids, suggesting that StARD1-mediated cholesterol trafficking to mitochondria is independent of MAM. TSPO, a protein particularly abundant in steroidogenic tissues and primarily localized in the mitochondrial outer membrane, has been suggested to play an important role in steroidogenesis via the transport of cholesterol to the mitochondrial inner membrane (IMM) [118, 119]. However, quite interestingly, recent studies using tissue-specific genetic deletion of TSPO demonstrated that TSPO is dispensable for steroidogenesis in Leydig cells [120], questioning the relevance of previous findings on TSPO using pharmacological ligands and inhibitors. These data underscore that TSPO does not play a significant role in the trafficking of cholesterol to IMM, and highlights the relevance of StARD1 in this process. Overall, these findings underscore the accumulation of cholesterol in mitochondrial membranes in patients and models of AD, and quite interestingly, paralell the increase in mitochondrial cholesterol observed in brain and liver mitochondria in NPC, arguing that this pool of cholesterol may be a common nexus in both AD and NPC.

5. Mitochondrial cholesterol promotes AD by depleting GSH

In addition to the amyloidogenic effect of cholesterol by fostering Aβ generation from APP, recent data has provided evidence that mitochondrial cholesterol accumulation sensitizes neurons to Aβ-induced neuroinflammation and neurotoxicity by depleting mGSH, effects that are prevented by mGSH replenishment [114, 116]. The mechanism of mitochondrial cholesterol accumulation involves the upregulation of StARD1 induced by Aβ *via* ER stress, confirming previous findings in hepatocytes [121]. Consistent wiht the reported increased expression of StARD1 in pyramidal hippocampal neurons of AD-affected patients, it is likely that this outcome may be accompanied by increased accumulation of cholesterol in mitochondria and subsequent depeltion of mGSH levels [117]. Moreover, a novel mouse model engineered to have enhanced cholesterol synthesis by SREBP-2 overexpression superimposed to APP/PS1 mutations triggered Aβ accumulation and tau pathology [122]. This triple transgenic model exhibited increased mitochondrial cholesterol loading and mGSH depletion and accelerated Aβ generation by β-secretase activation compared to APP/PS1 mice. Moreover, SREBP-2/APP/PS1 mice displayed synaptotoxicity, cognitive decline, tau hyperphosphorylation and neuro-fibrillary tangle formation in the absence of mutated tau, indicating that cholesterol, particularly mitochondrial cholesterol, can precipitate Aβ accumulation and tau pathology. Importantly, *in vivo* replenishment of mGSH with cell-permeable GSH monoethyl ester (GSH-EE) attenuated neuropathological features of AD in SREBP-2/APP/PS1 mice. These findings established that mitochondrial cholesterol promotes AD by selective depletion of mGSH stores. Therefore, understanding the molecular mechanisms on this cause-and-effect relationship may be of interest in AD.

The properties of GSH transport in isolated rat brain mitochondria appear to differ from those reported previously other tissues such as liver and kidney, as they were influenced most by inhibitors of the tricarboxylate carrier, citrate, isocitrate, and benzenyl-1,2,3-tricarboxylate [123] Moreover, in mouse brain mitochondria it has been shown that 2-oxoglutarate (OGC) and dicarboxylate (DIC) are both expressed in cortical neurons and astrocytes [124]. In addition, butylmalonate, an inhibitor of DIC, significantly decreased mGSH, suggesting DIC as an important GSH transporter in mouse cerebral cortical mitochondria. Interestingly, a role for UCP2 in the transport of mGSH has been described in neurons, suggesting that the transport of protons back into the matrix by UCP2 may favor the movement of GSH [125]. These studies suggest that multiple IMM anion transporters might be involved in mGSH transport and that they might differ in different cell populations within the brain. However, the fact that mitochondrial cholesterol loading selectively depleted mGSH indicated that this transport function is sensitive to cholesterol-mediated changes in membrane dynamics, similar to what has been reported in liver mitochondria. Indeed, the effect of cholesterol in the regulation of mGSH is mediated by the susceptibility of the OGC to perturbations in membrane dynamics. Functional expression analyses in Xenopus laevis oocytes microinjected with OGC cRNA showed enhanced transport of GSH in isolated mitochondria [126]. Moreover, cholesterol enrichment impairs the transport kinetics of 2-oxoglutarate via the OGC by decreasing mitochondrial membrane fluidity. Restoration of membrane dynamics by the fatty acid analog A_2C improves the activity of OGC and mGSH transport despite cholesterol enrichment. Therefore, strategies aimed to replenish mitochondrial membrane physical properties may be of relevance to AD by replenishing mGSH.

6. Regulation of mitochondrial cholesterol

The ER plays an essential role in the integration of multiple metabolic signals and the maintenance of cell homeostasis, particularly protein synthesis and folding. Under stress conditions induced by protein misfolding, the ER triggers an adaptive response called uncoupled protein response (UPR). To resolve ER stress, UPR promotes a decrease in protein synthesis, and an increase in protein degradation and chaperone production for protein folding. Aβ is well known to induce ER stress, which is believed to mediate in part the pathogenesis of AD [127]. Moreover, tauroursodeoxycholic acid (TUDCA), a chemical chaperone that prevents ER stress, has been shown to restore the mGSH pool in alcohol fed rats [128] and ameliorates alcohol-induced ER stress [121]. In line with these findings in liver, we have recently reported that TUDCA and PBA abolish Aβ-induced hepatic ER stress, mitochondrial cholesterol loading and subsequent mGSH depletion [116]. Emerging evidence has demonstrated that StARD1 is a previously unrecognized target of the UPR and ER stress signaling. Indeed, tunicamycin, an ER stress trigger, induces the expression of StARD1 in isolated hepatocytes and this effect is prevented by TUDCA treatment [121]. Moreover, mice fed a high cholesterol diet (HC) exhibited increased expression of StARD1. However, HC feeding downregulates the expression of SREBP-2-regulated target genes, including hydroxymethylglutaryl Co-A reductase, demonstrating that StARD1 is and an ER stress but not SREBP-2 regulated gene. In contrast to StARD1, the role of ER stress in the regulation of StART family members has been limited to StARD5 [129, 130], with conflicting results reported for StARD4 [130, 131]. As the UPR comprises three transducers, namely inositol requiring (IRE) 1α, PKR-like ER kinase (PERK), and activating transcription factor (ATF) 6α, which are controlled by the master regulator glucose-regulated protein 78 (GRP78 also known as BiP), further work is needed to examine the relative contribution of the involved arms of the UPR in the regulation of StARD1 by Aβ. Besides ER stress, StARD1 activation is regulated at the transcriptional and post-translational levels. In murine steroidogenic cells StARD1 activity and subsequent steroidogenesis increases upon StARD1 phosphorylation at serine residues [132, 133]. Whether or not StARD1 phosphorylation by Aβ regulates mitochondrial cholesterol homeostasis remains to be explored. If so, then the identification of putative kinases that phosphorylate and activate StARD1 may be of potential relevance in AD. The other unresolved question relates as to the mechanism whereby Aβ induces ER stress. As ER Ca^{2+} homeostasis is a key housekeeping mechanism to maintain ER function, it is conceivable that Aβ may disrupt ER Ca^{2+}, thereby causing ER stress. Whether Aβ modulates the activity of the ER Ca^{2+} pump SERCA, whose disruption is known to trigger ER stress remains to be investigated.

7. Concluding remarks

With an expected increase in cases, AD may represent one of the most important health burdens in the near future worlwide. Therefore the identification of effective therapeutic treatments for AD is of priority for health authorities around the world. Unfortunately our limited understanding of the molecular pathways underlying AD has curved the possibilities to have effective treatments at hand. While cholesterol and in particular hypercholesterolemia has been identified as a risk factor for AD development, the causal effect of cholesterol and the impact of cholesterol-lowering approach in AD still remains controversial. Unexpectedly, evidence in the last five years has indicated that the small pool of cholesterol in mitochondria plays an important role in AD, as its accumulation in mitochondria causes mGSH depletion amplifying the neurotoxic effects of Aβ peptides. Therefore, targeting mGSH may be of therapeutic relevance in AD. However, mGSH is regulated by its transport through mito-chondrial inner membrane via specific carriers that are sensitive to changes in mitochondrial membrane properties. Hence the mere increase in cytosolic GSH by GSH prodrugs, such as N-acetylcysteine, may not be effective in restoring mGSH as cytosolic GSH would not be transported into mitochndrial matrix due to cholesterol-mediated disruption in mitochondrial membrane dynamics. Thus, more specific approaches would imply the use of membrane-permeable GSH prodrugs such as GSH ethyl ester, which has been shown to protect against AD in experimental models and is known to cross the BBB. Alternatively, targeting the increase in mitochondrial cholesterol by antagonizing StARD1 may arise as another attractive possiblity in the future. This approach requires a better understanding of the cell biology of StARD1 and in the identification of BBB permeable specific StARD1inhibitors. We are looking forward to these and other more exciting discoveries to start controlling the onset and progression of this devastating disease.

Acknowledgements

This chapter is dedicated to the many patients, past and present that suffer AD, and very especially to my mother.

The work was supported by CIBEREHD, Fundació la Marató de TV3 and Grants PI11/0325 (META) from the Instituto de Salud Carlos III and Grant SAF2012-34831 from Plan Nacional de I+D, Spain; and the Center Grant P50-AA-11999 (Research Center for Liver and Pancreatic Diseases) funded by NIAAA/NIH. I want to thank the people in my lab who have made major contributions to unveil the role of mitochondrial cholesterol in Alzheimer, in particular Drs. Anna Fernandez, Carmen Garcia-Ruiz, Elisabet Barbero-Camps and Anna Colell.

Author details

José C. Fernández-Checa[1,2,3]

Address all correspondence to: checa229@yahoo.com

1 Department of Cell Death and Proliferation, Instituto Investigaciones Biomedicas de Barcelona, CSIC, Barcelona, and Liver Unit-Hospital Clinic-IDIBAPS, Spain

2 Centro de Investigación Biomédica en Red (CIBERehd), Barcelona, Spain

3 University of Southern California Research Center for Alcohol Liver and Pancreatic Diseases and Cirrhosis, Keck School of Medicine, USC, Los Angeles, CA, USA

References

[1] Katzov H, Chalmers K, Palmgren J, Andreasen N, Johansson B, Cairns NJ et al (2004) Genetic variants of ABCA1 modify Alz- heimer disease risk and quantitative traits related to beta-amyloid metabolism. Hum Mutat 23(4):358–367

[2] Whitehouse PJ (1997) Genesis of Alzheimer's disease. Neurology 48(5 Suppl 7):S2–S7

[3] Selkoe, D.J. 2001. Alzheimer's disease: genes, proteins, and therapy. Physiol. Rev. 81(2): 741–766.

[4] Cummings JL (2004) Alzheimer's disease. N Engl J Med 351 (1):56–67

[5] Bertram L, Tanzi RE (2005) The genetic epidemiology of neuro- degenerative disease. J Clin Invest 115(6):1449–1457

[6] Minati, L., Edginton, T., Grazia Bruzzone, M., and Giaccone, G. 2009. Current concepts in Alzheimer's disease: a multidisciplinary review. Am. J. Alzheimers Dis. Other Demen. 24(2): 95–121.

[7] Bertram L, McQueen MB, Mullin K, Blacker D, Tanzi RE (2007) Systematic meta-analyses of Alzheimer disease genetic associa- tion studies: the AlzGene database. Nat Genet 39(1):17–23

[8] Holmes C (2002) Genotype and phenotype in Alzheimer's disease. Br J Psychiatry 180:131–134

[9] St George-Hyslop PH, Petit A (2005) Molecular biology and genetics of Alzheimer's disease. C R Biol 328(2):119–130

[10] Tanzi RE, Bertram L (2005) Twenty years of the Alzheimer's disease amyloid hypothesis: a genetic perspective. Cell 120 (4):545–555

[11] Corder, E.H., Saunders, A.M., Strittmatter, W.J., Schmechel, D.E., Gaskell, P.C., Small, G.W., et al. 1993. Gene dose of apolipoprotein E type 4 allele and the risk of Alzheimer's disease in late onset families. Science, 261(5123): 921–923.

[12] Strittmatter, W.J., Saunders, A.M., Schmechel, D., Pericak-Vance, M., Enghild, J., Salvesen, G.S., and Roses, A.D. 1993. Apolipoprotein E: high-avidity binding to beta-amyloid and increased frequency of type 4 allele in late-onset familial Alzheimer disease. Proc. Natl. Acad. Sci. U.S.A. 90(5): 1977–1981.

[13] Poirier, J., Bertrand, P., Poirier, J., Kogan, S., Gauthier, S., Poirier, J., et al. 1993. Apolipoprotein E polymorphism and Alzheimer's disease. Lancet, 342(8873): 697–699.

[14] Chartier-Harlin, M.-C., Parfitt, M., Legrain, S., Pérez-Tur, J., Brousseau, T., Evans, A., et al. 1994. Apolipoprotein E, 3 4 allele as a major risk factor for sporadic early and late-onset forms of Alzheimer's disease: analysis of the 19q13.2 chromosomal region. Hum. Mol. Genet. 3(4): 569–574.

[15] Mendoza-Oliva A, Zepeda A, Arias C. The Complex Actions of Statins in Brain and their Relevance for Alzheimer's Disease Treatment: an Analytical Review. Curr Alzheimer Res. 2014 Oct 1

[16] Opie L.H. Can dementia be lessened by statins. The Lancet 384: 953, 2014.

[17] Hardy, J., and Allsop, D. 1991. Amyloid deposition as the central event in the aetiology of Alzheimer's disease. Trends Pharmacol. Sci. 12(10): 383–388.

[18] Hardy, J.A., and Higgins, G.A. 1992. Alzheimer's disease: the amyloid cascade hypothesis. Science, 256(5054): 184–185.

[19] Clippingdale AB, Wade JD, Barrow CJ (2001) The amyloid-beta peptide and its role in Alzheimer's disease. J Pept Sci 7(5):227–249

[20] Dickson DW (1997) The pathogenesis of senile plaques. J Neuro- pathol Exp Neurol 56(4):321–339

[21] Naslund J, Haroutunian V, Mohs R, Davis KL, Davies P, Greengard P et al (2000) Correlation between elevated levels of amyloid beta- peptide in the brain and cognitive decline. JAMA 283(12):1571– 1577

[22] Billings, L.M., Oddo, S., Green, K.N., McGaugh, J.L., and LaFerla, F.M. 2005. Intra-neuronal Ab causes the onset of early Alzheimer's disease-related cognitive deficits in transgenic mice. Neuron, 45 (5): 675–688.

[23] D'Andrea, M.R., Nagele, R.G., Wang, H.Y., Peterson, P.A., and Lee, D.H. 2001. Evidence that neurones accumulating amyloid can undergo lysis to form amyloid plaques in Alzheimer's disease. Histopathology, 38(2): 120–134.

[24] Gouras, G.K., Tsai, J., Naslund, J., Vincent, B., Edgar, M., Checler, F., et al. 2000. Intraneuronal Ab42 accumulation in human brain. Am. J. Pathol. 156(1): 15–20.

[25] Oddo, S., Caccamo, A., Shepherd, J.D., Murphy, M.P., Golde, T.E., Kayed, R., et al. 2003. Triple-transgenic model of Alzheimer's disease with plaques and tangles: intracellular Ab and synaptic dysfunction. Neuron, 39(3): 409–421.

[26] Wirths, O., Multhaup, G., and Bayer, T.A. 2004. A modified beta- amyloid hypothesis: intraneuronal accumulation of the beta- amyloid peptide–the first step of a fatal cascade. J. Neurochem. 91(3): 513–520.

[27] Glabe, C. 2001. Intracellular mechanisms of amyloid accumulation and pathogenesis in Alzheimer's disease. J. Mol. Neurosci. 17(2):137–145.

[28] Bahr, B.A., Hoffman, K.B., Yang, A.J., Hess, U.S., Glabe, C.G., and Lynch, G. 1998. Amyloid beta protein is internalized selectively by hippocampal field CA1 and causes neurons to accumulate amyloidogenic carboxyterminal fragments of the amyloid pre- cursor protein. J. Comp. Neurol. 397(1): 139–147.

[29] Friedrich, R.P., Tepper, K., Ronicke, R., Soom, M., Westermann, M., Reymann, K., et al. 2010. Mechanism of amyloid plaque formation suggests an intracellular basis of Ab pathogenicity. Proc. Natl. Acad. Sci. U.S.A. 107(5): 1942–1947.

[30] Rajendran, L., Honsho, M., Zahn, T.R., Keller, P., Geiger, K.D., Verkade, P., and Simons, K. 2006. Alzheimer's disease beta- amyloid peptides are released in association with exosomes. Proc. Natl. Acad. Sci. U.S.A. 103(30): 11172–11177.

[31] Busciglio, J., Pelsman, A., Wong, C., Pigino, G., Yuan, M., Mori, H., and Yankner, B.A. 2002. Altered metabolism of the amyloid beta precursor protein is associated with mitochondrial dysfunction in Down's syndrome. Neuron, 33(5): 677–688.

[32] Chui, D.H., Dobo, E., Makifuchi, T., Akiyama, H., Kawakatsu, S., Petit, A., et al. 2001. Apoptotic neurons in Alzheimer's disease frequently show intracellular Ab42 labeling. J. Alzheimers Dis. 3 (2): 231–239.

[33] Zhang, Y., McLaughlin, R., Goodyer, C., and LeBlanc, A. 2002. Selective cytotoxicity of intracellular amyloid beta peptide 1–42 through p53 and Bax in cultured primary human neurons. J. Cell Biol. 156(3): 519–529.

[34] Casas, C., Sergeant, N., Itier, J.M., Blanchard, V., Wirths, O., van der Kolk, N., et al. 2004. Massive CA1/2 neuronal loss with intraneuronal and N-terminal truncated Ab42 accumulation in a novel Alzheimer transgenic model. Am. J. Pathol. 165(4): 1289– 1300.

[35] LaFerla, F.M., Tinkle, B.T., Bieberich, C.J., Haudenschild, C.C., and Jay, G. 1995. The Alzheimer's Ab peptide induces neurodegenera- tion and apoptotic cell death in transgenic mice. Nat. Genet. 9(1): 21–30.

[36] Takahashi, R.H., Milner, T.A., Li, F., Nam, E.E., Edgar, M.A., Yamaguchi, H., et al. 2002. Intraneuronal Alzheimer Ab42 accumulates in multivesicular bodies and is associated with synaptic pathology. Am. J. Pathol. 161(5): 1869–1879.

[37] Almeida, C.G., Tampellini, D., Takahashi, R.H., Greengard, P., Lin, M.T., Snyder, E.M., and Gouras, G.K. 2005. Beta-amyloid accumulation in APP mutant neurons reduces PSD-95 and GluR1 in synapses. Neurobiol. Dis. 20(2): 187–198.

[38] Tampellini, D., Magrane, J., Takahashi, R.H., Li, F., Lin, M.T., Almeida, C.G., and Gouras, G.K. 2007. Internalized antibodies to the Ab domain of APP reduce neuronal Ab and protect against synaptic alterations. J. Biol. Chem. 282(26): 18895–18906.

[39] Jonsson, T., Atwal, J. K., Steinberg, S., Snaedal, J., Jonsson, P. V., Bjornsson, S., et al. (2012). A mutation in APP protects against Alzheimer's disease and age-related cognitive decline. *Nature* 488, 96–99.

[40] Hatami A, Albay R 3rd, Monjazeb S, Milton S, Glabe C., Monoclonal Antibodies Against Aβ42 Fibrils Distinguish Multiple Aggregation State Polymorphisms in vitro and in Alzheimer's Disease Brain. J.Biol. Chem, October 3 2014

[41] Haass, C. (2004). Take five – BACE and the gamma-secretase quartet con- duct Alzheimer's amyloid beta-peptide generation. *EMBO J.* 23, 483–488.

[42] Thathiah, A., Horre, K., Snellinx, A., Vandewyer, E., Huang, Y., Ciesielska, M., et al. (2013). beta-arrestin 2 regulates Abeta generation and gamma-secretase activity in Alzheimer's disease. *Nat. Med.* 19, 43–49.

[43] Hooper, N. M., and Turner, A. J. (2002). The search for alpha-secretase and its potential as a therapeutic approach to Alzheimer s disease. *Curr. Med. Chem.* 9, 1107–1119.

[44] Lin, M. T., and Beal, M. F. (2006). Alzheimer's APP mangles mitochondria. *Nat. Med.* 12, 1241–1243.

[45] Devi, L., Prabhu, B. M., Galati, D. F., Avadhani, N. G., and Anandatheerthavarada, H. K. (2006). Accumulation of amyloid precursor protein in the mitochondrial import channels of human Alzheimer's disease brain is associated with mitochon- drial dysfunction. *J. Neurosci.* 26, 9057–9068.

[46] Maxfield FR, Tabas I. Role of choleserol and lipid organization in disease. Nature 438:612-621, 2005.

[47] Goritz, C., Mauch, D.H., and Pfrieger, F.W. 2005. Multiple mechanisms mediate cholesterol-induced synaptogenesis in a CNS neuron. Mol. Cell. Neurosci. 29(2): 190–201.

[48] Pfrieger, F.W. 2003. Cholesterol homeostasis and function in neurons of the central nervous system. Cell. Mol. Life Sci. 60(6): 1158– 1171.

[49] Thiele, C., Hannah, M.J., Fahrenholz, F., and Huttner, W.B.2000. Cholesterol binds to synaptophysin and is required for biogenesis of synaptic vesicles. Nat. Cell Biol.2(1): 42–49.

[50] Sparks DL, Scheff SW, Hunsaker JC 3rd, Liu H, Landers T, Gross DR. Induction of Alzheimer-like beta-amyloid immunoreactivity in the brains of rabbits with dietary cholesterol.Exp Neurol. 1994 Mar;126(1):88-94

[51] Refolo LM, Malester B, LaFrancois J, Bryant-Thomas T, Wang R, Tint GS, Sambamurti K, Duff K, Pappolla MA. Hypercholesterolemia accelerates the Alzheimer's amyloid pathology in a transgenic mouse model.Neurobiol Dis. 2000 Aug;7(4):321-31

[52] Thirumangalakudi L, Prakasam A, Zhang R, Bimonte-Nelson H, Sambamurti K, Kindy MS, Bhat NR. High cholesterol-induced neuroinflammation and amyloid precursor protein processing correlate with loss of working memory in mice.J Neurochem. 2008 Jul;106(1):475-85.

[53] Oksman M, Iivonen H, Hogyes E, Amtul Z, Penke B, Leenders I, Broersen L, Lütjohann D, Hartmann T, Tanila H. Impact of different saturated fatty acid, polyunsaturated fatty acid and cholesterol containing diets on beta-amyloid accumulation in APP/PS1 transgenic mice. Neurobiol Dis. 2006 Sep;23(3):563-72.

[54] Shie FS, Jin LW, Cook DG, Leverenz JB, LeBoeuf RC. Diet-induced hypercholesterolemia enhances brain A beta accumulation in transgenic mice.Neuroreport. 2002 Mar 25;13(4):455-9

[55] Levin-Allerhand JA, Lominska CE, Smith JD. Increased amyloid- levels in APPSWE transgenic mice treated chronically with a physiological high-fat high-cholesterol diet.J Nutr Health Aging. 2002;6(5):315-9.

[56] Ujiie M, Dickstein DL, Carlow DA, Jefferies WA. Blood-brain barrier permeability precedes senile plaque formation in an Alzheimer disease model. Microcirculation. 2003 Dec;10(6):463-70.

[57] Winkler EA, Sagare AP, Zlokovic BV. The pericyte: a forgotten cell type with important implications for Alzheimer's disease? Brain Pathol. 2014 Jul;24(4):371-86

[58] Wahrle, S., Das, P., Nyborg, A.C., McLendon, C., Shoji, M., Kawarabayashi, T., et al. 2002. Cholesterol-dependent gamma- secretase activity in buoyant cholesterol-rich membrane micro- domains. Neurobiol. Dis. 9(1): 11–23.

[59] Vetrivel, K.S., and Thinakaran, G. 2010. Membrane rafts in Alzheimer's disease beta-amyloid production. Biochim. Biophys. Acta, 1801(8): 860–867.

[60] Anstey, K. J., Lipnicki, D. M., and Low, L. F. (2008). Cholesterol as a risk factor for dementia and cognitive decline: a systematic review of prospec- tive studies with meta-analysis. *Am. J. Geriatr. Psychiatry* 16, 343–354.

[61] Notkola, I. L., Sulkava, R., Pekkanen, J., Erkinjuntti, T., Ehnholm, C., Kivinen, P., et al. (1998). Serum total cholesterol, apolipoprotein E epsilon 4 allele, and Alzheimer's disease. *Neuroepidemiology* 17, 14–20.

[62] Wolozin, B., Kellman, W., Ruosseau, P., Celesia, G. G., and Siegel, G. (2000). De- creased prevalence of Alzheimer disease associated with 3-hydroxy- 3-methyglutaryl coenzyme A reductase inhibitors. *Arch. Neurol.* 57, 1439–1443.

[63] Martins, I.J., Berger, T., Sharman, M.J., Verdile, G., Fuller, S.J., and Martins, R.N. 2009. Cholesterol metabolism and transport in the pathogenesis of Alzheimer's dis- ease. J. Neurochem. 111(6): 1275– 1308.

[64] Burns MP, Igbavboa U, Wang L, Wood WG, Duff K. Cholesterol distribution, not to- tal levels, correlate with altered amyloid precursor protein processing in statin-treat- ed mice. Neuromolecular Med. 2006;8(3):319-28

[65] Chan SL, Kim WS, Kwok JB, Hill AF, Cappai R, Rye KA, Garner B. ATP-binding cas- sette transporter A7 regulates processing of amyloid precursor protein in vitro. J Neurochem. 2008 Jul;106(2):793-804.

[66] Kim WS, Weickert CS, Garner B. Role of ATP-binding cassette transporters in brain lipid transport and neurological disease. J Neurochem. 2008 Mar;104(5):1145-66.

[67] DiPaolo G, Kim TW. Linking lipids to Alzheimer's disease: cholesterol and beyond. Nat Rev Neurosci. 2011 May;12(5):284-96

[68] Urano Y, Ochiai S, Noguchi N. Suppression of amyloid-β production by 24S-hydrox- ycholesterol via inhibition of intracellular amyloid precursor protein trafficking. FA- SEB J. 2013 Oct;27(10):4305-15.

[69] Eckert GP, Cairns NJ, Maras A, Gattaz WF, Müller WE. Cholesterol modulates the membrane-disordering effects of beta-amyloid peptides in the hippocampus: specific changes in Alzheimer's disease. Dement Geriatr Cogn Disord. 2000 Jul-Aug;11(4): 181-6.

[70] Mason RP, Shoemaker WJ, Shajenko L, Chambers TE, Herbette LG. Evidence for changes in the Alzheimer's disease brain cortical membrane structure mediated by cholesterol. Neurobiol Aging. 1992 May-Jun;13(3):413-9.

[71] Heverin M, Bogdanovic N, Lütjohann D, Bayer T, Pikuleva I, Bretillon L, Diczfalusy U, Winblad B, Björkhem I. Changes in the levels of cerebral and extracerebral sterols in the brain of patients with Alzheimer's disease. J Lipid Res 2004 Jan;45(1):186-93.

[72] Sparks DL. Coronary artery disease, hypertension, ApoE, and cholesterol: a link to Alzheimer's disease? Ann N Y Acad Sci. 1997 Sep 26;826:128-46.

[73] Abad-Rodriguez J, Ledesma MD, Craessaerts K, Perga S, Medina M, Delacourte A, Dingwall C, De Strooper B, Dotti CG. Neuronal membrane cholesterol loss enhances amyloid peptide generation. J Cell Biol. 2004 Dec 6;167(5):953-60.

[74] Ledesma MD, Abad-Rodriguez J, Galvan C, Biondi E, Navarro P, Delacourte A, Dingwall C, Dotti CG. Raft disorganization leads to reduced plasmin activity in Alzheimer's disease brains. EMBO Rep. 2003 Dec;4(12):1190-6.

[75] Cole SL, Grudzien A, Manhart IO, Kelly BL, Oakley H, Vassar R. Statins cause intracellular accumulation of amyloid precursor protein, beta-secretase-cleaved fragments, and amyloid beta-peptide via an isoprenoid-dependent mechanism. J Biol Chem. 2005 May 13;280(19):18755-70.

[76] Li G, Higdon R, Kukull WA, Peskind E, Van Valen Moore K, Tsuang D, van Belle G, McCormick W, Bowen JD, Teri L, Schellenberg GD, Larson EB. Statin therapy and risk of dementia in the elderly: a community-based prospective cohort study. Neurology. 2004 Nov 9;63(9):1624-8.

[77] Rea TD, Breitner JC, Psaty BM, Fitzpatrick AL, Lopez OL, Newman AB, Hazzard WR, Zandi PP, Burke GL, Lyketsos CG, Bernick C, Kuller LH. Statin use and the risk of incident dementia: the Cardiovascular Health Study.Arch Neurol. 2005 Jul;62(7): 1047-51.

[78] Zandi PP, Sparks DL, Khachaturian AS, Tschanz J, Norton M, Steinberg M, Welsh-Bohmer KA, Breitner JC; Cache County Study investigators. Do statins reduce risk of incident dementia and Alzheimer disease? The Cache County Study. Arch Gen Psychiatry. 2005 Feb;62(2):217-24.

[79] Carlsson CM, Gleason CE, Hess TM, Moreland KA, Blazel HM, Koscik RL, Schreiber NT, Johnson SC, Atwood CS, Puglielli L, Hermann BP, McBride PE, Stein JH, Sager MA, Asthana S. Effects of simvastatin on cerebrospinal fluid biomarkers and cognition in middle-aged adults at risk for Alzheimer's disease. J Alzheimers Dis. 2008 Mar;13(2):187-97.

[80] Hoglund K, Thelen KM, Syversen S, Sjogren M, von Bergmann K, Wallin A, Vanmechelen E, Vanderstichele H, Lutjohann D, Blennow K. The effect of simvastatin treatment on the amyloid precursor protein and brain cholesterol metabolism in patients with Alzheimer's disease. Dement Geriatr Cogn Disord. 2005;19(5-6):256-65.

[81] Riekse RG, Li G, Petrie EC, Leverenz JB, Vavrek D, Vuletic S, Albers JJ, Montine TJ, Lee VM, Lee M, Seubert P, Galasko D, Schellenberg GD, Hazzard WR, Peskind ER. Effect of statins on Alzheimer's disease biomarkers in cerebrospinal fluid. J Alzheimers Dis. 2006 Dec;10(4):399-406.

[82] Posse de Chaves E. Reciprocal regulation of cholesterol and beta amyloid at the subcellular level in Alzheimer's disease. Can J Physiol Pharmacol 90: 753-764, 2012.

[83] Mohamed A, Saavedra L, Di Pardo A, Sipione S, Posse de Chaves E. β-amyloid inhibits protein prenylation and induces cholesterol sequestration by impairing SREBP-2 cleavage. J Neurosci. 2012 May 9;32(19):6490-500.

[84] Bjorkhem I, Meaney S (2004) Brain cholesterol: long secret life behind a barrier. Arterioscler Thromb Vasc Biol 24(5):806–815

[85] Dietschy JM, Turley SD (2004) Thematic review series: brain Lipids. Cholesterol metabolism in the central nervous system during early development and in the mature animal. J Lipid Res 45(8):1375–1397

[86] Goldstein JL, DeBose-Boyd RA, Brown MS. Protein sensors for membrane sterols. Cell. 2006 Jan 13;124(1):35-46

[87] Jo Y, DeBose-Boyd RA. Control of cholesterol synthesis through regulated ER-associated degradation of HMG CoA reductase. Crit Rev Biochem Mol Biol. 2010 Jun;45(3): 185-98.

[88] Pfrieger FW. Cholesterol homeostasis and function in neurons of the central nervous system.Cell Mol Life Sci. 2003 Jun;60(6):1158-71.

[89] Jurevics H, Morell P. Cholesterol for synthesis of myelin is made locally, not imported into brain. J Neurochem 64: 895-901, 1995.

[90] Wahrle SE, Jiang H, Parsadanian M, Legleiter J, Han X, Fryer JD, Kowalewski T, Holtzman DM. ABCA1 is required for normal central nervous system ApoE levels and for lipidation of astrocyte-secreted apoE. J Biol Chem. 2004 Sep 24;279(39): 40987-93.

[91] Karten B, Campenot RB, Vance DE, Vance JE. Expression of ABCG1, but not ABCA1, correlates with cholesterol release by cerebellar astroglia. J Biol Chem. 2006 Feb 17;281(7):4049-57

[92] Herz J. Apolipoprotein E receptors in the nervous system. Curr Opin Lipidol. 2009 Jun;20(3):190-6.

[93] Poirier J. Apolipoprotein E and cholesterol metabolism in the pathogenesis and treatment of Alzheimer's disease.Trends Mol Med. 2003 Mar;9(3):94-101.

[94] Puglielli L, Konopka G, Pack-Chung E, Ingano LA, Berezovska O, Hyman BT, Chang TY, Tanzi RE, Kovacs DM. Acyl-coenzyme A: cholesterol acyltransferase modulates the generation of the amyloid beta-peptide. Nat Cell Biol. 2001 Oct;3(10):905-12.

[95] Bogdanovic N, Bretillon L, Lund EG, Diczfalusy U, Lannfelt L, Winblad B, Russell DW, Björkhem I. On the turnover of brain cholesterol in patients with Alzheimer's disease. Abnormal induction of the cholesterol-catabolic enzyme CYP46 in glial cells. Neurosci Lett. 2001 Nov 13;314(1-2):45-8.

[96] Lung EG, Guileyardo JM, Rusell DW. cDNA cloning of cholesterol 24-hydroxylase, a mediator of cholesterol homeostasis in the brain. Proc Natl Acad Sci. USA 96: 7238-43, 1999.

[97] Lund EG, Xie C, Kotti T, Turley SD, Dietschy JM, Russell DW. Knockout of the cholesterol 24-hydroxylase gene in mice reveals a brain-specific mechanism of cholesterol turnover. J Biol Chem. 2003 Jun 20;278(25):22980-8.

[98] Kim WS, Rahmanto AS, Kamili A, Rye KA, Guillemin GJ, Gelissen IC, Jessup W, Hill AF, Garner B.Role of ABCG1 and ABCA1 in regulation of neuronal cholesterol efflux to apolipoprotein E discs and suppression of amyloid-beta peptide generation. J Biol Chem 282: 2851-2861, 2007.

[99] Muscat GE, Wagner BL, Hou J, Tangirala RK, Bischoff ED, Rohde P, Petrowski M, Li J, Shao G, Macondray G, Schulman IG. Regulation of cholesterol homeostasis and lipid metabolism in skeletal muscle by liver X receptors.J Biol Chem. 2002 Oct 25;277(43):40722-8.

[100] Whitney KD, Watson MA, Collins JL, Benson WG, Stone TM, Numerick MJ, Tippin TK, Wilson JG, Winegar DA, Kliewer SA. Regulation of cholesterol homeostasis by the liver X receptors in the central nervous system. Mol Endocrinol. 2002 Jun;16(6): 1378-85.

[101] Eckert GP, Vardanian L, Rebeck GW, Burns MP. Regulation of central nervous system cholesterol homeostasis by the liver X receptor agonist TO-901317. Neurosci Lett. 2007 Aug 9;423(1):47-52.

[102] Burns MP, Rebeck GW. Intracellular cholesterol homeostasis and amyloid precursor protein processing. Biochim Biophys Acta 1801: 853-859, 2010.

[103] Burns M, Gaynor K, Olm V, Mercken M, LaFrancois J, Wang L, Mathews PM, Noble W, Matsuoka Y, Duff K. Presenilin redistribution associated with aberrant cholesterol transport enhances beta-amyloid production in vivo. J Neurosci. 2003 Jul 2;23(13): 5645-9.

[104] Jin LW, Shie FS, Maezawa I, Vincent I, Bird T. Intracellular accumulation of amyloidogenic fragments of amyloid-beta precursor protein in neurons with Niemann-Pick type C defects is associated with endosomal abnormalities. Am J Pathol. 2004 Mar; 164(3):975-85.

[105] Runz H, Rietdorf J, Tomic I, M Bernard, Byereuthe K, Pepperkok R, Hartmann T. Inhibition of intracellular cholesterol transport alters presenilin localization and amyloid precursor protein processing in neuronal cells. J Neurosci 22: 1679-1689.

[106] Kågedal K, Kim WS, Appelqvist H, Chan S, Cheng D, Agholme L, Barnham K, McCann H, Halliday G, Garner B. Increased expression of the lysosomal cholesterol transporter NPC1 in Alzheimer's disease. Biochim Biophys Acta. 2010 Aug;1801(8): 831-8.

[107] Caglayan S, Takagi-Niidome S, Liao F, Carlo AS, Schmidt V, Burgert T, Kitago Y, Füchtbauer EM, Füchtbauer A, Holtzman DM, Takagi J, Willnow TE. Lysosomal sorting of amyloid-β by the SORLA receptor is impaired by a familial Alzheimer's disease mutation. Sci Transl Med. 2014 Feb 12;6(223):223ra20.

[108] Fucho R, Martínez L, Baulies A, Torres S, Tarrats N, Fernandez A, Ribas V, Astudillo AM, Balsinde J, Garcia-Rovés P, Elena M, Bergheim I, Lotersztajn S, Trautwein C, Appelqvist H, Paton AW, Paton JC, Czaja MJ, Kaplowitz N, Fernandez-Checa JC, García-Ruiz C. ASMase regulates autophagy and lysosomal membrane permeabilization and its inhibition prevents early stage non-alcoholic steatohepatitis. J Hepatol. 2014 Nov;61(5):1126-34.

[109] Karaca I, Tamboli IY, Glebov K, Richter J, Fell LH, Grimm MO, Haupenthal VJ, Hartmann T, Gräler MH, van Echten-Deckert G, Walter J. Deficiency of sphingosine-1-phosphate lyase impairs lysosomal metabolism of the amyloid precursor protein. J Biol Chem. 2014 Jun 13;289(24):16761-72.

[110] Van Echten-Deckert G, Walter J. Sphingolipids: critical players in Alzheimer's disease. Prog Lipid Res 51: 378-93, 2012.

[111] Garcia-Ruiz C, Mari M, Colell A, Morales A, Montero J, Terrones O, Basañez G, Fernandez-Checa JC Mitochondrial cholesterol in health and disease. Histol Histopathol 24: 117-32, 2009

[112] Bosch M, Marí M, Herms A, Fernández A, Fajardo A, Kassan A, Giralt A, Colell A, Balgoma D, Barbero E, González-Moreno E, Matias N, Tebar F, Balsinde J, Camps M, Enrich C, Gross SP, García-Ruiz C, Pérez-Navarro E, Fernández-Checa JC, Pol A. Caveolin-1 deficiency causes cholesterol-dependent mitochondrial dysfunction and apoptotic susceptibility. Curr Biol. 2011 Apr 26;21(8):681-6.

[113] Colell A, Fernández A, Fernández-Checa JC. Mitochondria, cholesterol and amyloid beta peptide: a dangerous trio in Alzheimer disease. J Bioenerg Biomembr. 2009 Oct; 41(5):417-23.

[114] Fernandez A, Llacuna L, Fernandez-Checa JC, Colell A. Mitochondrial cholesterol loading exacerbates amyloid beta peptide-induced inflamation and neurotoxicity. J Neurosci 2009; 29: 6394-405.

[115] Caron KM, Soo SC, Wetsel WC, Stocco DM, Clark BJ, Parker KL. argeted disruption of the mouse gene encoding steroidogenic acute regulatory protein provides insights into congenital lipoid adrenal hyperplasia. Proc Natl Acad Sci U S A. 1997 Oct 14;94(21):11540-5.

[116] Barbero-Camps E, Fernández A, Baulies A, Martinez L, Fernández-Checa JC, Colell A. Endoplasmic reticulum stress mediates amyloid β neurotoxicity via mitochondrial cholesterol trafficking. Am J Pathol. 2014 Jul;184(7):2066-81.

[117] Webber KM, Stocco DM, Casadesus G, Bowen RL, Atwood CS, Previll LA, Harris PL, Zhu X, Perry G, Smith MA. Steroidogenic acute regulatory protein (StAR): evidence

of gonadotropin-induced steroidogenesis in Alzheimer disease. Mol Neurodegener 1:14, 2006.

[118]   Papadopoulos, V., and Miller, W. L. (2012). Role of mitochondria in steroido- genesis. *Best Pract. Res. Clin. Endocrinol. Metab.* 26, 771–790.

[119]   Miller, W. L. (2013). Steroid hormone synthesis in mitochondria. *Mol. Cell. Endocrinol.* 379, 62–73.

[120]   Morohaku, K., Pelton, S. H., Daugherty, D. J., Butler, W. R., Deng, W., and Selvaraj, V. (2014). Translocator protein/peripheral benzodiazepine receptor is not required for steroid hormone biosynthesis. *Endocrinology* 155, 89–97.

[121]   Fernandez A, Matias N, Fucho R, Ribas V, Von Montfort C, Nuño N, Baulies A, Martinez L, Tarrats N, Mari M, Colell A, Morales A, Dubuquoy L, Mathurin P, Bataller R, Caballeria J, Elena M, Balsinde J, Kaplowitz N, Garcia-Ruiz C, Fernandez-Checa JC. ASMase is required for chronic alcohol induced hepatic endoplasmic reticulum stress and mitochondrial cholesterol loading. J Hepatol. 2013 Oct;59(4):805-13.

[122]   Barbero-Camps E, Fernández A, Martínez L, Fernández-Checa JC, Colell A. APP/PS1 mice overexpressing SREBP-2 exhibit combined Aβ accumulation and tau pathology underlying Alzheimer's disease. Hum Mol Genet. 2013 Sep 1;22(17):3460-76.

[123]   Wadey, A. L., Muyderman, H., Kwek, P. T., and Sims, N. R. (2009). Mitochon- drial glutathione uptake: characterization in isolated brain mitochondria and astrocytes in culture. *J. Neurochem.* 109(Suppl. 1), 101–108.

[124]   Kamga, C. K., Zhang, S. X., and Wang, Y. (2010). Dicarboxylate carrier-mediated glutathione transport is essential for reactive oxygen species homeostasis and normal respiration in rat brain mitochondria. *Am. J. Physiol. Cell Physiol.* 299, C497–C505.

[125]   de Bilbao, F., Arsenijevic, D., Vallet, P., Hjelle, O. P., Ottersen, O. P., Bouras, C., etal. (2004). Resistance to cerebral ischemic injury in UCP2 knockout mice: evidence for a role of UCP2 as a regulator of mitochondrial glutathione levels. *J. Neurochem.* 89, 1283–1292.

[126]   O. Coll, A. Colell, C. García-Ruiz, N. Kaplowitz, J.C. Fernández-Checa. Sensitivity of the 2-oxoglutarate carrier to alcohol intake contributes to mitochondrial glutathione depletion. Hepatology, 38 (2003), pp. 692–702

[127]   Ferreiro E, Resende R, Costa R, Oliveira CR, Pereira CM. An endoplasmic-reticulum-specific apoptotic pathway is involved in prion and amyloid-beta peptides neurotoxicity. Neurobiol Dis. 2006 Sep;23(3):669-78.

[128]   Colell A, Coll O, García-Ruiz C, París R, Tiribelli C, Kaplowitz N, Fernández-Checa JC. Tauroursodeoxycholic acid protects hepatocytes from ethanol-fed rats against tumor necrosis factor-induced cell death by replenishing mitochondrial glutathione. Hepatology. 2001 Nov;34(5):964-71.

[129] R.E. Soccio, R.M. Adams, K.N. Maxwell, J.L. Breslow, Differential gene regulation of StarD4 and StarD5 cholesterol transfer proteins. Activation of StarD4 by sterol regulatory element-binding protein-2 and StarD5 by endoplasmic reticulum stress, J. Biol. Chem. 280 (2005) 19410–19418.

[130] D. Rodriguez-Agudo, M. Calderon-Dominguez, M.A. Medina, S. Ren, G. Gil, W. M. Pandak, ER stress increases StarD5 expression by stabilizing its mRNA and leads to relocalization of its protein from the nucleus to the membranes, J. Lipid Res. 53 (2012) 2708–2715.

[131] S. Yamada, T. Yamaguchi, A. Hosoda, T. Iwawaki, K. Kohno, Regulation of human STARD4 gene expression under endoplasmic reticulum stress, Biochem. Biophys. Res. Commun. 343 (2006) 1079–1085.

[132] P.R. Manna, J.W. Soh, D.M. Stocco, The involvement of specific PKC iso- enzymes in phorbol ester-mediated regulation of steroidogenic acute reg- ulatory protein expression and steroid synthesis in mouse Leydig cells, Endocrinology 152 (2011) 313–325.

[133] F. Arakane, S.R. King, Y. Du, C.B. Kallen, L.P. Walsh, H. Watari, D.M. Stocco, J. F. Strauss, Phosphorylation of steroidogenic acute regulatory protein (StAR) modulates its steroidogenic activity, J. Biol. Chem. 272 (1997) 32656–32662.

4

Genetic, Biochemical and Histopathological Aspects of Familiar Alzheimer's Disease

Genaro Gabriel Ortiz, Fermín P. Pacheco-Moisés,
Erika D. González-Renovato, Luis Figuera,
Miguel A. Macías-Islas, Mario Mireles-Ramírez,
L. Javier Flores-Alvarado, Angélica Sánchez-López,
Dhea G. Nuño-Penilla, Irma E. Velázquez- Brizuela,
Juan P. Sánchez-Luna and Alfredo Célis de la Rosa

Additional information is available at the end of the chapter

1. Introduction

Alzheimer's disease (AD) is the most common cause of dementia among people over 65 years. In industrialized countries it is the fourth leading cause of death; in our country and although there are no figures on the epidemiological dimension of this disease, statistical projections of Latin American countries with similar socio-economic conditions, estimated to affect approximately 350,000 Mexicans. This disease is slowly progressive and is characterized by progressive dementia with profound memory loss, decreased ability to perform routine tasks, difficulties in judgment, disorientation, personality changes, difficulty in learning, and loss of language skills. On average, its duration is 8-12 years in which there is a period of 2-3 years when the symptoms are very subtle and often goes unnoticed. Although protocols have carefully designed clinical diagnosis, diagnostic certainty of Alzheimer's disease is about 85% and it was confirmed by post-mortem brain examination.

The EA is inseparably between clinical symptoms of dementia and the presence of specific lesions in selected areas of the cerebral cortex and hippocampus. The neuropathological findings in the disease exhibited protein deposits manifest as neuritic plaques; consisting of extracellular deposits composed of amyloid β (β-amyloid plaques). Also showed neurofibrillary interneuronal tangles consisting of cytoskeletal protein tau, and granulo-vaculoar degeneration (figures 6-9), reduction and dysfunction of synapses, neuronal death and reduction in overall brain volume. AD typically affects the hippocampus and adjacent structures, memory deficits are typically among the earliest and most pronounced signs of AD. When pathological changes spread beyond the hippocampus, other cognitive areas also become affected [1-5]

It is possible to distinguish two different types of AD based upon age onset and familial aggregation: familiar AD (FAD) and late-onset AD (LOAD). FAD is characterized by Mendelian inheritance (autosomal dominant) and early onset (<60 years). FAD represents about 5–10% of all AD cases [5], LOAD is characterized by later onset >60 years) and complex patterns of inheritance. Although they differ in age onset, both forms of the disease are defined by the same pathological features; neuronal loss and the presence of beta-amyloid plaques and neurofibrillary tangles (figure 6, 7). Plaques are extracellular deposits of insoluble amyloid proteins while tangles are intracellular aggregations of hyperphosphorilated tau protein. AD has a characteristic onset, is very gradual and insidious, this is a particularity that distinguishes the pathology from other forms of dementia [9].

Genetic factors, including risk factors are related to AD. In a minority of hereditary disease appears so in a pattern of autosomal dominant inheritance. Chromosomes 21, 14 and 1 are associated with some familial forms of early onset; Moreover, the late-onset familial forms appear linked to chromosomes 12 and 19. Sporadic cases, most cannot be explained from a genetic point of view, although they have stated hypotheses that the action of toxic agents or unidentified infectious affecting genetic aspects (figure 1) [9-11].

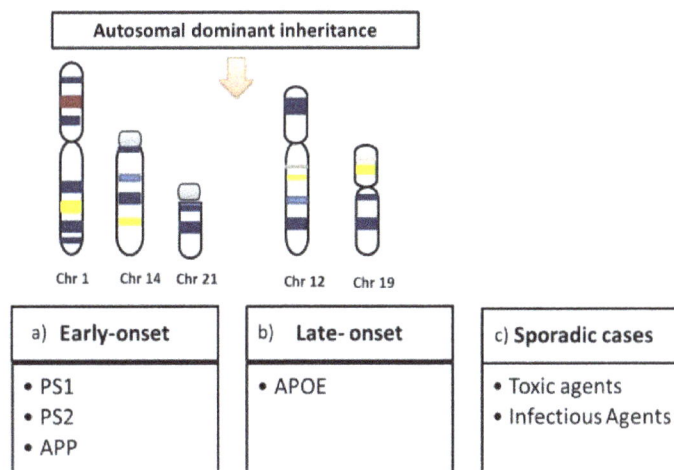

Figure 1. Genetic Factors Related to Alzheimer's Dementia

Genetic factors related to Alzheimer's dementia.

a. Chromosomes 1, 14 and 21 are associated with Early-onset forms. These genes are linked to mutations on Presenilin-1 (PS1), Presenilin-2 (PS2) and Amiloid precursor protein (APP), numerous studies has demonstrated that changes in these proteins predisposes individuals to familial Alzheimer disease.

b.   Chromosomes 14 and 19 are associated with late-onset forms. Chromosome 19 are linked to mutations on Apolipoprotein E, specially isoform 4 (APOE4)

c.   Others form Of Alzheimer's dementia cannot be explained from a genetic point of view, including sporadic cases [11-13].

Mutations in different genes located on chromosomes 14 and 1, responsible for the disease of early onset familial Alzheimer (EOAD), in a portion of patients show penetrance (proportion of individuals that show the phenotype) about 100 % with autosomal dominant inheritance. In the EOAD, autosomal dominant mutations in three genes; APP encoding amyloid precursor protein, PSEN1 and PSEN2 encoding presenilin 1 and 2, lead to increased production of beta amyloid [8]. The presenilin mutations, especially PS1 (~85%), are much more common in early onset familial AD than APP mutation [14]. It has demonstrated the existence of a locus on chromosome 14 (14q 24.3) in a group of families with EOAD. Using positional cloning the gene designated S 182, which contains 14 exons and encodes the synthesis of a protein of 467 amino acids (aa) called presenilin 1 (PS-1) (figure 1) containing from 6 to 9 transmembrane domains, and two hydrophilic regions was isolated that are oriented towards the cytosol; at least over 90 different mutations found in the gene of the PS-1 to chromosome 14 mutations (include: His163Arg, Ala246Glu, Leu286Val and Cys410Tyr) most display complete penetrance, but a common mutation is Glu318Gly and this predisposes individuals to familial Alzheimer disease. All except one are missense and represent about 30-50% of cases of EAFP. PSEN-1 mutations are usually associated with very aggressive EOAD, with duration of dementia of about 5 years [6]. PSEN-2 gene mutations are very rare. The ages at onset of EOAD are thought to vary (PSEN-1 25–60, APP 40–65 and PSEN-2 45–84. It is quite possible that other genes with mutations leading to EOAD will be found [14-18].

The first gene associated with late forms family was identified in a family sample by applying a new method of genetic analysis. The identified Apo E locus is located on the long arm of chromosome 19 (figure 2).

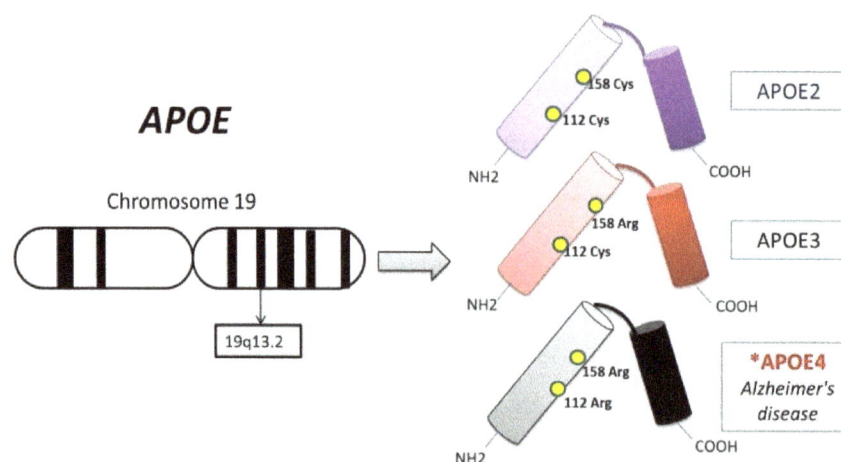

Figure 2. Association Between Apo E Isoforms and Alzheimer's Disease

The *APOE* gene is located on the long arm of **chromosome 19** at position 13.2. There are 3 different alleles of the *APOE* gene, producing 3 major isoforms, Known as *ApoE2* (cys112, cys158), *ApoE3* (cys112, arg158), and *ApoE4* (arg112, arg158). The APOE4 isoform of increases an individual's risk for developing late-onset Alzheimer disease [19,20].

Numerous studies have reported association between Apo E (locus) and EOAD, and sporadic cases. The relationship between Apo E and AD is set by the overrepresentation of one of the common protein isoforms in the group of patients. Of the 3 major isoforms, known as E2, E3 and E4, E4 are frequently associated with the onset of the disease [19]. The hypothesis of the existence of a locus that could explain some of the cases EOAD was confirmed in 1992, in which several groups pre-sented evidence of a locus on chromosome 14; this was named, along with S 182, PS-1 or AD3. The role of the PS-1 gene in the body is unknown. Homology with family proteins Notch/lin-12 indicates that it may play an important role in signal transduction, and it is stated that the process involved in apoptosis. The gene of the PS-1 is expressed in different regions of the brain, skeletal muscle, kidney, pancreas, placenta and heart. Processing produces two fragments, this process occurs naturally and is under control. An increase of the amount of PS-1 produced by the cells, *in vitro*, is not accompanied by increase in the concentration of the fragments. Of the 10 exons which holds the PS-1 gene, most of the mutations are linked to exon 5 (comprising the transmembrane domain 1 and 2) and exon 8 (comprising the trans-membrane domain 6 and 7). The effects on the PS-1 gene, in the 2 sites mentioned above, show a significant difference with respect to age at onset of the disease when compared to each other. Patients with mutations in the transmembrane domain (TD) 6 and 7, having an average age of onset higher than those with mutations in the DT 1 and 2.14 [12,13]

All mutations, except one, are missense, resulting in a change of one aa by another. The mutation known as D9 is one of the exceptions, and described in many families of diverse origin (English, Japanese, Australian, Latin's). Involvement cause removal of exon 9, the reading frame is not altered processing and disposal site and the corresponding fragments. The mutation has the remarkable feature that is expressed in almost all families, spastic paraparesia; a phenotype that does not seem to occur with any other mutation. In an English family mutation was detected in codon 141 of the PS-1 gene with incomplete penetrance. The involvement was manifested in a change of Iso by Val, the disease started with an average age of onset of 55 years. The muta-tions cause about 2% of all EOEA, and occur less frequently than those found in the PS-1 gene. Only found two missense mutations with incomplete penetrance [12].

Another gene, called STM-2, was isolated families descendants of German settlers installed in the Volga region in Russia. The STM-2 gene encodes a 448 aa protein called presenilin 2 (PS-2), PS-2 contained 12 exons, 10 of which were coding exons, and that the primary transcript encodes a 448 amino acid polypeptide with 67 (80%) of homology to PS1 gene in some regions. This protein has been identified as part of the enzymatic complex that cleaves amyloid beta peptide from APP. The affected families had a missense mutation at codon 141, resulting in a change of aspartic (Asp) by Iso. In these families had been excluded linkage to chromosomes 14 and 21. The PS-2 gene also contains 12 exons, and the protein for which it encodes contains from 6 to 9 DT [12,13].

The PS-2 transmembrane protein has 67% homology to the sequence of aa from the PS-1, and therefore depending homology. The PS-2 is localized in the endoplasmic reticulum with the hydrophilic domains oriented towards the cytoplasm (figure 3).

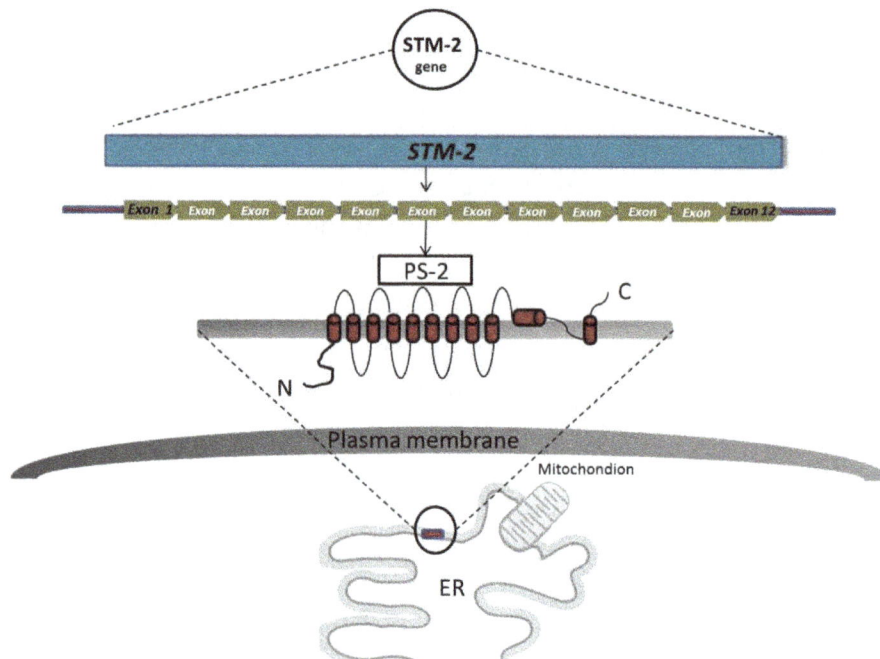

Figure 3. The Membrane Topology of PS2

The PS-2 protein is derived from the STM-2 gene from 12 exons. The ten-transmembrane-domain model of PS2 with one hydrophobic region and 10 associated to the membrane of the endoplasmic reticulum.

The homology between PS-1 and PS-2 is particularly focused on the DT. The amino-terminal domain and the domain located between exons 8 and 10, have the lowest degree of homology and are supposed to be where the functional specificity of each of the proteins resides. Another mutation that is associated with EOEA is located at codon 239 and is manifested in a change of methionine (Met) by Val. As can be seen, the mutation sites are different from those presented in the PS-1, characterized by incomplete penetrance. It is thought that mutations in the gene of the PS-2 may cause an increase in apoptotic activity and consequently accelerating the process of neurodegeneration. In EOEA families with mutations in the PS-1 gene the average age of onset is much younger (45 years, range 29 to 62 years) that family with mutations in the PS-2 gene (52 years, range between 40 and 88 years).

Neuritic plaques, extracellular structures observable in AD are composed of amyloid beta peptide (ßA) and other elements such as glia and astrocytes (figures 6-9). The main constituent is ßA peptide natural product of the metabolism of amyloid precursor protein (APP). The study of families in the Volga allowed to demonstrate that the total amount of long ßA peptide (aa 42-43) and short (39-40 aa) were significantly lower in the case of mutations in the PS-2 gene mutations compared the PS-1 gene. Experiments *in vivo* have suggested that the PS-1 mutant altered proteolytic processing of APP at the C-terminal peptide SSA to favor deposition ßA long peptide (more insoluble and form faster kinetic characteristics). The relationship between PS-1 and EA does not seem clear; however, studies from fibroblasts and plasma from patients who have inherited mutations in this gene, demonstrating that the effect of these changes is to increase the ßA 42 peptide in the plasma. The mechanism by which PS-1 exerts its effect in AD is unknown. Mutations in the protein produce the same effect as the effects on the PPA. Presenilins are involved indirectly with a gamma-secretase, an enzymatic complex that processes of the PPA, and may be triggering or mediating its activity (figure 4) [12,13].

The presence of extracellular amyloid-peptide-containing neuritic plaques and intracellular neurofibrillary tangles and the loss of synapses in defined regions of the brain are the hallmarks associated with both familial and sporadic AD postmortem pathology.

In this chapter we reviewed the genetic, molecular, biochemical, and histopathological aspects of familiar AD (EOAD) linked to chromosomes 1, 14 and 19 and especially those found in a region of the state of Jalisco, Mexico.

2. Detection of EOAD

Detect EOAD is more complicated than LOAD [9], as their main symptom not always starts with memory loss, but with other symptoms such as vision problems, motor or speech, mood swings, irritability, disorientation even in familiar places, difficulty in learning and reasoning, lack of initiative and isolation. People who have it take longer and be diagnosed, as some of these symptoms are related to stress or depression. Early of AD detection is very important for the patient. Family environment can accelerate disease because the stress, is misunderstanding, lack of patience, affected by worsening symptoms, while good weather and a quiet home life makes slow the progression of symptoms (figure 5). Family members who have been able to detect early Alzheimer's must be psychologically and emotionally prepared to live with the disease [21-23].

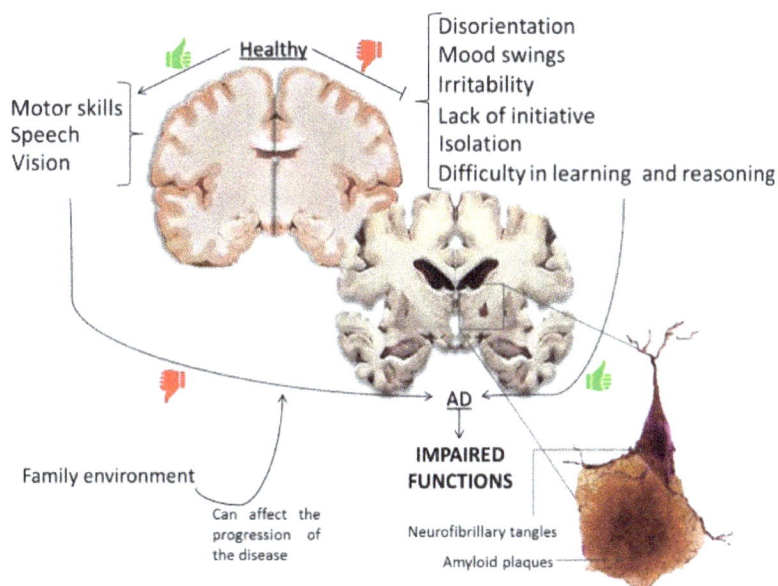

Figure 4. Symptomatology in Alzheimer´s Disease *versus* Helathy Control

During the initial stage, clinical data are diverse, but can be mentioned as the most significant: progressive memory loss, and changes in personality and behavior. Another common finding in EOAD is language difficulty (aphasia) such as naming which is commonly detected my persons close to the patients. Common findings that develop by the progression of AD are depression, headaches, seizures, myoclunus, Babinsky reflex, grasp reflex, extra-pyramidal signs and Parkinsonism. Being a progressive disease, the disease is progressive, and clinical signs and symptoms may vary from patient to patient; also the evolution of a patient with EOAD has been studied, it is believed that there are differences according between FAD and non NFAD; that patients with FAD compared to NFAD presented more frequent non-memory symptoms like visuospatial deficit. FAD present more memory deficit tan NFAD at the moment of the initial clinic visit. FAD has more tendencies to develop more headaches, myoclonus, gait abnormalities and pseudobulbar affect. Healthy control presents unaltered motor skills, speech and vision functions. However, in Alzheimer's Disease patient's motor skills, speech and vision functions are impaired, while disorientation, mood swings, irritability, lack of initiative, isolation and difficulty in learning and reasoning is also present. On the other hand family environment can affect the progression of the symptomatology of the disease.

The age of onset difference between FAD and NFAD is that FAD develops 14 years earlier and the MMSE score is lower than NFAD. Initial clinic visits from patients with cognitive deterioration are to be focused on the disease onset, course and symptoms. A powerful tool for the clinical insight is the Mini- Mental State Examination (MMSE) which will help to know the cognitive status of the individual (Screening). There modifying factors that have been related to the progression of AD like is the level of school attendance, history of headaches and seizures. Now a day it is important to follow the guidelines to pursue a genetic testing of the most common mutations in AD allowing clinicians evaluate and manage patients with early onset dementias.

3. Risk factors in early life

The risk of dementia and Alzheimer's disease starts from the maternal womb. Fetal malnutrition, low birth weight and not breastfeeding may have long-term negative consequences. It has been shown that these and other conditions related to the early age of life, increased susceptibility to several chronic diseases, particularly cardiovascular disease and its risk factors (e.g. hyperinsulinemia, diabetes, atherosclerosis, hypertension, lipid disorders). The socioeconomic conditions are associated with other handicaps: nutrition, environmental stimulation, access to education, neuron-developmental, body growth, and subsequent cognitive performance. Several studies have used anthropometric as height indices, the length of the leg and arm, head circumference as markers of neurodevelopment in the first years of life and have found an inverse association with dementia and AD in later life.

The educational attainment has been the most studied factor. In most studies, low educational attainment is associated consistently with increased risk of cognitive impairment and dementia. There are multiple explanations for the association between low IQ and dementia:

1. Education produces a selection bias, since people with more education may show better performance on cognitive tests

2. Education is associated with other factors such as socioeconomic status early age, nutrition, IQ and adult life as an occupation, health and better lifestyles

3. Education increases cognitive reserve offering a potentiating neuroprotection and inducing long term [11-13].

4. Genetics and Alzheimer

Some genes were associated with AD: on chromosome 21 gene encoding the β-amyloid precursor protein, on chromosome 14 gene presenilin 1 (PS1), on the chromosome 1 gene for presenilin 2 (PS2), on chromosome 17 gene coding for protein, and chromosome 19 in the apolipoprotein E (ApoE). Four alleles of ApoE, which is believed to play an important role in AD is the ApoE type 4 are known ApoE4 allele has been seen as a risk factor for AD, with an attributable risk estimated 45 to 60%. Thus the approach to the diagnosis of probable AD also includes the study of ApoE.

Mutations in different genes located on chromosomes 14 and 1, responsible for EOAD of, in a portion of patients show a penetration (proportion of individuals that show the phenotype) about 100% with autosomal dominant. It has demonstrated the existence of a locus on chromosome 14 (14q 24.3) in a group of families with EOAD. Using the positional cloning the gene designated S 182, which contains 14 exons and encodes the synthesis of a protein of 467 amino acids (aa) called presenilin 1 (PS-1) containing from 6 to 9 transmembrane domains and two hydrophilic regions was isolated that are oriented towards cytosol [5,6] [table 1].

4.1. The Amyloid Precursor Protein (APP)

The amyloid precursor protein is a member of a family to understand her two similar proteins, APLP1 and APLP2. The APP is present in dendrites, cell bodies and axons of neurons and neuronal function is unknown. APP is synthesized in the rough endoplasmic reticulum, Golgi glycosylated and released into the membrane as a transmembrane protein, leaving the portion containing 613-671 β amyloid partially included in the membrane. The APP gene is located on chromosome 21; several investigators have identified many families of patients in whom the disease is declared prematurely, mutations in the APP gene located in different parts of the same: thus, a Swedish family found a double mutation at codons 670 and 671, and in other families, a mutation at codon 717 is detected. In these families, only those who show these mutations suffer from Alzheimer's disease, which proves without any doubt that there is a relationship between APP metabolism and Alzheimer's disease. The APP can experience a different metabolism to generate as a final product or other fragments. In the non-amyloidogenic pathway, APP secretase short region within the amyloid form a COOH-terminal 83 amino acid residues or appas called fragment CT83. In the amyloidogenic pathway, two enzymes called β-secretase or BACE and γ-secretase cleaved APP at the N terminal of the peptide sequence in endosomal compartments Aß, while the γ -secretase cleaves the C-terminal sequence ab on cell surface or near it. Two types of γ -secretase that are called presenilin-1 and presenilin-2: PS1 and PS1. These enzymes are currently the subject of extensive studies, because its blockade by drugs theoretically decrease the formation of β-amyloid [14, 15].

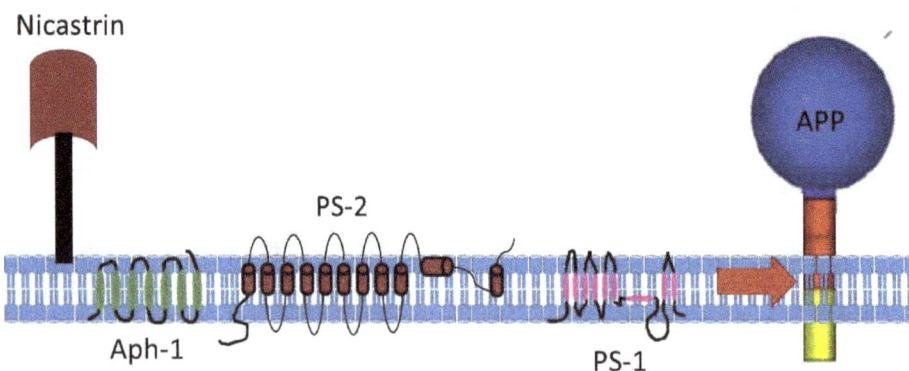

Figure 5. γ – Secretase Complex

The γ-secretase complex is composed of four membrane proteins: nicastrin, aph-1, PS-2, and presenilin (1 or 2). The actual catalytic site is in presenilin. Cleavage of APP and other substrates occurs in the membrane. Presenilins are involved indirectly with the complex.

More than 90 different mutations have been found in the gene for the PS-1 on chromosome 14. All mutations but one are missense and represent about 30-50% of cases of another gene, in this case located on chromosome 1 was found was using the same strategy that isolated the PS-1. Gene, called STM-2, was isolated families descended from German settlers installed in the Volga region in Russia (ref). STM-2 gene encodes a 448 aa protein called presenilin 2 (PS-2), named after the latter has homology (over 80%) compared to the PS-1 gene in some regions (ref.). The mutations cause about 2% of total EOAD and occur less frequently than those found in the PS-1 gene. Only found two missense mutations penetrance incomplete [16].

The first gene associated with late forms family was identified in a family sample by applying a new method of genetic analysis. The identified Apo E locus is located on the long arm of chromosome 19. Numerous studies have reported association between Apo E (locus) and EOAD, and sporadic cases. The relationship between Apo E and EA is set by the over-representation of one common protein isoforms in the group of patients. Of the 3 major isoforms, known as E2, E3 and E4, E4 is often found associated with the appearance of the disease [13].

This table exhibited examples of some important mutations per gene; number of gene mutations identified are also shown in table.

Mutations in PSEN1 gene				
Number of Mutations in gene	Mutations	Exon/Domain	Onset	General description of Clinical data
185 mutations described in 405 families	Thr116Asn	5/ HL-I	Early Autosomal dominant heritance	
	Met139Val	5/ TM-II		
	Met146Leu	5/ TM-II		
	Thr291Pro	9/ HL-VI (MA)		
	Leu171Pro	6/ TM-III		
	Ala431Glu	12/ HL-VIII		
Mutations in PSEN2 gene				
Number of Mutations in gene	Mutations	Exon/Domain	Onset	
13 mutationes describen in 22 families	Ala85Val	4/ N-term	Early Autosomal dominant heritance	• Progressive memory loss • Changes in personality and behavior. • Language difficulty • Depression • Headaches • Seizures • Myoclunus • Babinsk reflex • Grasp reflex • Cerebellar signs
	Thr122Pro	5/ HL-1		
	Thr122Arg	5/ HL-1		
	Ser130Leu	5/ HL-1		
	Asn141Ile	5/ TM-II		
	Val148Ile	5/ TM-II		
Mutations in APP gene				
Number of Mutations in gene	Mutations	Exon/Domain	Onset	
33 mutations described in 90 families	Ala692Gly	17/ N-term	Late	
	Glu693Gln	17/ N-term		
	Ile716Phe	17/ TM-I		
	Val717Leu	17/ TM-I		
	Leu723Pro	17/ TM-I		
	Ile716Val	17/ TM-I		
Mutations in APOe gene				
Number of Mutations in gene	Mutations	Exon/Domain	Onset	
88 mutations described	-293 (G/T)	Promoter region	Late	
	-427 (T/C)	Promoter region		
	-491 (A/T)	Promoter region		

Table 1. Mutations

4.2. Presenilin (PS-1 and PS-2)

The hypothesis of the existence of a locus that could explain some of the cases EAFP was confirmed in 1992, in which several groups pre-sat evidence of a locus on chromosome 14; this was named, along with S 182, PS-1 or AD3. The role of the PS-1 gene in the organism is unknown. Its homology to proteins of the Notch / lin-12 family suggests that it may play a role in signal transduction, and it is stated that the process involved in gene apoptosis. The PS-1 is expressed in different regions of brain, skeletal muscle, kidney, pancreas, placenta and the heart. Its processing produces 2 fragments, this process occurs naturally and is under control. An increase of the amount of PS-1 produced by the cells, *in vitro*, is not accompanied by increase in the concentration of the fragments. Of the 14 exons which holds the PS-1 gene, most of the mutations are linked to exon 5 (comprising the transmembrane domain 1 and 2) and exon 8 (comprising the transmembrane domain 6 and 7); the effects on the PS-1 gene, in the 2 sites mentioned above show a significant difference with respect to age at onset of the disease when compared to each other, patients with mutations in the transmembrane domain (DT) 6 and 7, with a mean age of onset higher than those with mutations in the DT 1 and 2 [16-17].

All mutations, except one, are missense, resulting in a change of a from one another. The mutation known as D9 is one of the exceptions, and described in many families of diverse origin (English, Japanese, Australian and Latin´s). Involvement causes the elimination of exon 9 (the deletion occurs); do not changes the reading frame processing and disposal site and the corresponding fragments. The mutation has the remarkable feature that is expressed in almost all families, spastic paraparesy, and a phenotype that is not apparent with any other mutation. In an England family a mutation was detected in codon 141 of PS-1 gene with incomplete penetrance. The involvement is manifested in a change of Iso by Val, the disease began with an average age of onset of 55 years [16-17].

The STM 2 gene (located on chromosome 1), also known as AD 4, PS-2, the affected families had a missense mutation at codon 141, resulting in a change of aspartic acid (Asp) by Iso. In these families ligations were excluded chromosomes 14 and 21. The PS-2 gene also contains 10 exons, and the protein for which it encodes contains 6 to 9 DT. The PS-2 transmembrane protein has 67% homology to the sequence of aa from the PS-1, and therefore, the homology in función. PS-2 is localized in the endoplasmic reticulum with the hydrophilic domains oriented cytoplasm. The homology between PS-1 and PS-2 is particularly focused on the DT. The amino-terminal domain and the domain located between exons 8 and 10, has the lowest degree of homology and which is supposed to be the functional specificity of each of the living proteins (ref.). Another mutation that is associated with the EOAD is located at codon 239 and is manifested in a change of methionine (Met) to Valina (Val) (ref.). As can be seen, the mutation sites are different from those presented in the PS-1, characterized by a penetration incomplete. This data support that mutations in the gene of the PS-2 cause an increase in apoptotic activity, and therefore accelerate neurodegeneration.

In EOAD families with mutations in the PS-1 gene the average age of onset is much younger (45 years, range 29 to 62 years) that families with mutations in the PS-2 gene (52 years, range between 40 and 88 years) (ref.).

Senile plaques, extracellular structures observable in AD, are formed by the amyloid beta peptide (ßA) and other elements such as glia and astrocytes. The main constituent is ßA peptide natural product of the metabolism of amyloid precursor protein (APP) (Figure 7). The study of families in the Volga possible to show that the total amount of long ßA peptide (aa 42-43) and short (39-40 aa) were significantly lower in the case of mutations in the PS-2 gene mutations compared in PS-1 (figure2) Gene *in vivo* experiments have suggested that the mutated PS-1 alters the proteolytic processing of APP at the C-terminal peptide ßA to favor the deposition of peptide ßA long (more insoluble form and kinetic properties more fast), the relationship between PS-1 and EA does not seem clear; however, studies from fibroblasts and plasma from patients with inherited mutations in this gene, show that the effect of these changes is to increase the peptide ßA 42 in plasma. The mechanism by the that PS-1 exerts its effect in AD; mutations in the protein produce the same effect that the damages in the PPA. Presenilins are involved in an indirect way with gama-secretase, an enzyme that processes of the PPA. The PS-2 mutated gene causes the disease, and also makes it through the common mechanism to which reference was made earlier, that is, increasing the concentration of peptide ßA 42. Transgenic animals carrying the PS-1 mutation, have 2 times ßA peptide 42 in the brain tissue compared to normal mice. Although mutations in the APP gene and the PS-1 and PS-2 genes have a dramatic effect, they are only responsible for 50% of cases of EOAD. They represent 5% of all cases in the general population. Men and women who inherit two copies (one from each parent) of the gene, called ApoE4, are at very high risk of developing Alzheimer. However, the two copies of ApoE4 is rare, affecting only 2 percent of the population, while about 15 percent of people carry a single copy of this version of the gene. This gene affects a protein involved in the transport of cholesterol in cholesterol-the cells is a crucial component of all cell membranes, including nerve cells. Nerve cells are constantly responding to experience, through the development, improvement, reduction or elimination of their electrochemical contact with other nerve cells. For all these processes, efficient transport of cholesterol is critical. Only about 10-15 percent of the population carries one copy of E4, over 50 percent of people who develop Alzheimer's disease are carriers E4. However, the increased risk of E4 seems confined largely to women.

Functional magnetic resonance imaging was used to examine the connections in the network of the brain's memory and has been shown that in older women with the E4 variant, this network of interconnected brain regions which usually share a synchronized pattern activity-shows a loss of sync, a pattern typically seen in Alzheimer's patients. In healthy elderly women (but not men) with at least one E4 allele, activity in a brain area called precuneus seems out of sync with other regions whose activation patterns in general are closely coordinated

We performed genetic and Spanish-language neuropsychological control; Mexican persons without dementia known to be at 50% risk of inheriting one of two *PSEN1* mutations. Early declines in performance on the Trail Making Test, delayed recall of a 10-word list, the Wechsler Adult Intelligence Scale Block Design Test, and total MMSE score in these subjects. In a previous work (ref) we explore the sub-items on the MMSE that best differentiate *PSEN1* mutation carriers (MCs) and non-carriers (NCs) and explore the relationship of age and education to these scores. Neuropsicological data exhibited MCs performed worse than NCs on the Mini-Mental State Examination. In multiple linear regression analyses a question frequently asked is: if APOE4 carriers had different results in function evaluations affected by

Alzheimer's disease, including episodic memory, working memory, mental speed, reaction time and vocabulary reading. As expected, performance in all tests (except for reading vocabulary, which tends to stay with age) declined by age groups, a sign of normal cognitive aging. But the APOE4 did not affect performance, indicating that people with APOE4 age normally in those cognitive functions, at least between 20 and 64 years old. According to the researchers, this finding suggests that APOE4 increases the risk of Alzheimer's later in life by an unknown process that accelerates or intensifies normal cognitive changes [24-27].

4.3. Beta-Amyloid (Aß)

Discovered in 1984 by Glenner et al., Is a peptide of 39-42 amino acids originating from the called amyloid precursor protein (APP) by the action of peptidadas called secretases. There are two major types of b-amyloid called amyloid-b and b-amyloid 1-40 1-42 according to the number of amino acids present. APP is a transmembrane protein having 770 aminácidos and located on different cell types. On its extracellular portion, the APP has several regions with neurotrophic activity.

Senile plaques in the brain parenchyma and vessel amyloid deposits are composed primarily amyloid beta peptide (Aß). Although the accumulation of Aß is common in non-demented elderly individuals in EA this accumulation is usually higher and / or faster. Currently, genetic evidence, in vitro experiments and in animal models suggest that the accumulation of brain Aß oligomers as might be an important development factor cognitivo deterioration; hence the removal of Aß in the brain is one of the therapeutic strategies for AD currently undergoing clinical trial. Aß is one of the normal internal proteolysis products transmembrane protein called APP (amyloid precursor protein). Excessive accumulation of Aß in AD could be explained by several mechanisms, some of them converging. Include increased production of Aß, kinetics of aggregation or self-assembly and quick removal of faulty brain as a result of: 1 an abnormally slow transport from the interstitial fluid into the cerebral spinal fluid (perivascular drainage) or plasma (transport through capillaries) and 2 deficiente proteolytic degradation. Excess production or the greater tendency of Aß oligomerization may explain the rapid deposition of Aß in some rare hereditary forms of AD, caused by mutations in APP or presenilin genes called 1 and 2, components of the secretase complex responsible for the generation of Aß. Instead, poor elimination could be relevant in the normal brain aging and may be magnified in the most common forms of AD called sporadic. Beyond a well-defined, as the inheritance of one or two e4 alleles of apolipoprotein E, a risk factor for sporadic AD probably has multiple risk factors include head trauma, ischemic events, hypertension, insulin resistance, among others, and a complex pathogenesis that is still far from being understood [14-15].

4.4. Tau protein

Tau belongs to the family of microtubule-associated proteins (MAPs) and normally binds to and stabilizes microtubules (MTs) in neurons. Tau protein has four different domains: the N-terminal, the proline rich, the microtubule-binding and the C-terminal domain. In the adult human brain six tau isoforms are expressed by different splicing of the same tau mRNA; they vary in the number of microtubule-binding domains (having either three or four) and in the number and size of N-terminal inserts [2]. Tau can be post-translationally modified in several ways (e.g. glycosylation, ubiquitination and oxidation), but phosphorylation is by far the most extensively studied and is paramount to AD pathology [2,3]. Hyperphosphorylation of tau especially on Ser214 and Ser262, leads to lose its ability to bind to MTs and may also sequester normal tau, preventing binding to MTs, resulting in disruption of the MT [4]. Hyperphosphorylated tau is also more resistant to proteases and this makes it more prone to aggregate to form PHFs in NFT´s. Neurofibrillary tangles (NFT) (figure 6) are one of the main diagnostic criteria of AD. Each of these lesions contains filamentous aggregates composed of the microtubule-associated protein (MAP) tau [9]. The normal function of tau protein is to stabilize axonal microtubules and regulate intracellular vesicle transport. Hyperphosphorylation of tau associated with AD impairs its ability to regulate microtubule assembly and promotes the protein aggregation into paired helical filaments (PHF). To understand the roles of normal and abnormal tau protein has been important to elucidate the structure and the mechanisms by which self-assembles it. Contains six human tau isoforms that result from splicing process ("splicing") alternative. The C-terminal domain containing 3 or 4 repetitive sequences involved in the binding of tau to microtubules that are key to the ability to promote their assembly One reason why a change in the functionality of tau is phosphorylation significant abnormal sites in their structure, essentially residues Ser/Thr Pro followed: Ser202, Thr205, Ser396 and Ser404 (22). Such phosphorylations are catalyzed by two protein kinases: the cdk5 / p35 and GSK3b system (32). In the cytoplasm, there is normally phosphorylated tau and it is postulated that these post-translational modifications regulate tau's ability to associate with microtubules and other cytoskeletal filaments. In AD, tau is hyperphosphorylated in these key sites, which changes the dynamics of action in regulating the interaction patterns within the cytoskeleton causing their self-association and training, progressively, PHF

No tau mutations have been reported to cause AD, but differences in tau haplotype and mutations may be the cause of other neurodegenerative disorders such as progressive supranuclear palsy [10]. NFT pathology in the brain occurs in a sequential manner. The altered protein Tau is less able to bind to other cytoskeletal proteins and added in lethal NFT seen in degenerating neurons of AD patients. The total length of p35 is normally regulated and has a very short half-life; degradation is usually carried out by its association with Cdk35, which the hyperphosphorylated. Moreover, p25 is completely stable, it accumulates in large amounts in EA (10 to 40 times and in the same regions where present NFT; levels Cdk5 and p35 have to remain stable in EA), maintains a permanent activation of Cdk5 and seems to precede the formation of NFTs. The connection between p25 and the formation of amyloid plaques is unknown. These findings provide several future therapeutic strategies: altered level of cut (cleavage) of p35, inhibition/blocking Cdk5 (necessary for day to day neuronal enzymes), blocking p25 or protease that produces it. Other proteins (protein associated with the cytoskeleton, focal adhesion kinase, glutaredoxin, utropina) have been implicated as mediators in the formation of NFTs or degeneration of neurons affected. The presence of few neurofibrillary tangles in the hippocampus and in the parahippocampal gyrus (in AD their presence is most notable in the entorhinal cortex) and senile plaques.

The possible role of Tau in dementia took center stage in AD with the discovery of mutations in the tau gene on chromosome 17; frontotemporal call Ademencia with Parkinsonism linked to chromosome 17 "(FTDP-17) includes a large number of mutations, which can result in a variety of currently known. These include fronto-temporal dementia (characterized by frontal and anterior temporal atrophy), Pick's disease (characterized by intra-neuronal inclusions called Pick bodies, Alternative Predominant in Clew of AD (AD @ AVPO-characterized by the lack of plates. presence of tangles predominantly in limbic and paralimbic cortical areas), progressive supranuclear palsy and corticobasal degeneration The shape of the Tau inclusions (including PH-Tau) depends partly on the causative mutation thereof; and those related to the PH-Tau inclusions produced in one or more anatomical sites from the cerebral cortex to the spinal cord, also Tau deposits can be found in neurons, tangles, Pick bodies or glial cells. The absence of plates, particularly of compact manifold, in many of the tauopathies suggests that Tau abnormalities are responsible for dementing disorder, including some variations of AD (e.g., AD-VPO). Known mutations occur in a reduced protein Tau Tau ability to interact with microtubules on production or Tau isoforms with four repeated microtubules together. These lead to the assembly of the Tau in similar or identical to those found in AD filaments. Several missense mutations also have a stimulating effect on filament formation heparin-induced Tau. The assembly of tau into filaments may be a gain of toxic function believed to be the underlying cause of death of nerve cells affected.[8].

4.5. Apo-E

Apolipoprotein E (ApoE) is the major apolipoprotein present in high-density lipoproteins (HDL) and is synthesized in the brain, primarily by astrocytes and to a lesser degree by microglia. ApoE is a 299 amino acid glycoprotein which organize into 2 functional domains; residues 1-191 form the amino-terminal (ApoE NT) "receptor binding domain" and residues 216-299 form the carboxyl-terminal (ApoE CT) "lipid binding domain". Both domains have been reported to be involved in the interaction between ApoE and Aβ. Three common isoforms of apoE exist in humans and result from amino acid interchanges at positions 112 and 158. ApoE2 has cysteines while apoE4 has arginines at both sites. ApoE3 has a cysteine and an arginine at positions 112 and 158, respectively. The most common form of apoE is apoE3, which is present in 77% of the general population; ~15% of the population have apoE4, and ~8% have the apoE2 [27]. The APOE ε4 allele markedly increases AD risk and decreases age of onset, likely through its strong effect on the accumulation of amyloid-β (Aβ) peptide. In contrast, the APOE ε2 allele appears to decrease AD risk [28]. ApoE4 is associated with an early age of AD onset. [29].

ApoE isoform differentially affect the apoE:lipid ratio of glia-secreted particles where apoE4 exhibits a higher apoE:lipid ratio compared to apoE3. ApoE mediates transport of glia-secreted particles to neurons for development, axon myelination, synaptogenesis and maintenance. Additionally, apoE redistributes cholesterol released after neuron injury or degeneration for membrane repair and remyelination [30]. The higher apoE:lipid ratio in apoE4 suggests that at similar apoE protein concentration, apoE4 may deliver less cholesterol to neurons, compared to apoE3. ApoE4 particles were also shown to be less efficient at inducing cholesterol efflux from neuronal cells compared to apoE3 [3l]. Brain apoE particles exhibit differing binding affinities to the amyloid-β peptide in a manner that is apoE isoform-dependent, therefore,

ApoE isoform may influence AD pathogenesis via direct or indirect interactions with Aβ. Furhermore, ApoE plays essential role in facilitating the proteolytic clearance of soluble Aβ. E4 apolipoprotein E isoform has been considered a risk factor for developing Alzheimer's disease. The exact mechanism by which the presence ApoE affects Alzheimer's is still unknown; appears to promote the formation and stabilizes the aggregation of beta amyloid fibril in plaques that appear in Alzheimer's disease. Aβ protein is considered the major component of these plates and is a proteolytic product of the precursor protein of Aβ peptide. The gene encoding apolipoprotein E (ApoE) is known as allelic variants APOEε2, and APOEε4 APOEε3 and a rare allelic variant known as APOEε3r APOEε3. In studies in populations of individuals with Alzheimer's disease and race from different geographical origins, it has been shown that APOEε4 allele is a risk factor that influences age of onset of symptoms. The APOEε4 allele is 50% of individuals with Alzheimer's disease and delayed onset of the presence of a copy of the allele increases the risk of late onset and three times in two copies in 12 times. Individuals with late onset carrying one or two copies of allele APOEε4 develop symptoms of disease 10 to 20 years earlier, compared with individuals not carrying this allele. The APOEε2, much less common in individuals with Alzheimer's disease and in the general population, allele appears to act as a protective factor for the onset of disease. The APOE-4 contributes to the accumulation of Aβ by slowing evacuation of the brain, which may explain why some people accumulate more Aβ, which other, increasing the risk of Alzheimer's. Individuals with APOE-e4 have much more protein Aβ in the brain, that individuals with the APOE-e2 and APOE-e3 (the other two common forms of protein gene) forms these data are obtained using the methodology of the microdialysis ; that involves the implantation of a dialysis membrane in a brain region to monitor chemical processes in the tissues of a living organism. [32-34].

5. Molecular markers for early Alzheimer's Disease

The rational approach of neurodegenerative diseases associated with dementia, particularly Alzheimer's disease, has led researchers around the world to think this entity as a systemic process that involves changes not only in the brain but also peripherally, so that has begun to seek so-called "peripheral biomarkers". These biomarkers can be found in platelets, lymphocytes, cultured fibroblasts and cerebrospinal fluid samples of patients affected [35]. Since AD has a long preclinical stage of the disease, the biomarker should also be predictive and. In AD, naturally, the biomarker should be relevantly linked to either amyloid- or tau pathology.

The hypothesis that the AD is systemic, has led to the search for peripherals markers, which can manifest biochemical changes related to the disease markers. Studies of the incidence and transmission patterns in families of patients with AD show that relatives of affected individuals have an increased risk of developing AD when compared with members of the general population. Concordance rates between monozygotic twins pro sides with EA are 40-60%, suggesting a strong but not absolute genetic influence of disease. Another significant problem is that some cognitively healthy subjects exhibit substantial AD type neuropathology [36]. On the other hand, some patients with severe cognitive impairment display very little neuropathology. It is also common that patients with other dementias, for example vascular dementia or dementia with Lewy bodies, have concomitant AD neuropathology or AD patients have vascular or LB pathology [37].

It has been hypothesized that the AD associated changes in CSF biomarkers would be evident before the clinical diagnosis of AD and could be used to predict the development of AD in MCI patients. For example, CSF Aβ42 levels were decreased and CSF tau and phospho tau levels were increased in those MCI patients who received a diagnosis of AD during a follow-up period of approximately four years [38].

Numerous different proteins and molecules that are present in CSF have been studied as potential biomarkers for AD, such as glycosylated acetylcholinesterase [39], transglutaminase [40], 24S-hydroxycholesterol [41], isoprostane [42]. It is also possible that the most accurate diagnosis of early AD can be achieved by using a panel of several different biomarkers [43]. Even though the above mentioned and numerous other molecules including neurofilament proteins, neuromodulin and neuronal thread protein have been studied [44], at the present, the only usable biomarkers are the CSF Aβ42, tau and phospho-tau levels in CSF.

Since platelets contain the amyloid precursor protein and secrete β-amyloid peptide, express neurotransmitters and some neuron-related proteins, such as NMDA receptors [45], in our group of work we are analyzing platelets from AD patients and subjects controls. Western blotting experiments of APP showed one protein of about 130 Kd and several proteins of about 106 to 110 Kd. The 130 Kd protein is the mature APP. The other proteins of lower molecular weights are the APP immature isoforms [46]. A high mature APP to immature APP isoform ratio (O.6 or higher) it has been related to a normal APP processing. Conversely, a lower ratio (< 0.6) it has been related to an altered APP processing [47]. We previously showed mature APP to immature APP isoform ratio in platelet samples of AD Mexican subjects was similar to the reported in previous studies [48]. This means that an increased degradation of this precursor protein is being performed in peripheral tissues. In addition, we found no statistical differences were detected for gender, age, and any specific ApoE allele in AD patients. Furthermore, statistical analysis between EOAD patients and LOAD suggests that no statistical differences among both groups in neither the APP isoforms nor any of the ApoE genotypes [46]. These data are in consonance with previous studies suggesting that ApoE genotyping is not sufficient as a diagnostic test for AD [49].

We have assessed the role of oxidative stress markers (lipoperoxides, nitric oxide metabolites) and membrane properties such as membrane fluidity in AD patients. We found a reduced fluidity in the platelet inner mitochondrial membrane in AD patients compared with healthy controls of similar age. It has been suggested that oxidative stress could be partially responsible for the diminution of membrane fluidity [50]. This change in membrane fluidity can modify the activities of the membrane-bound proteins such as transport or receptor proteins. At this regard, it has been hypothesized that a reduced fluidity of the inner mitochondrial membrane may diminish significantly the rate of mitochondrial ATP synthesis. Oxidative stress and mitochondrial failure has been associated to Alzheimer's pathology [51]. We measured the rate of mitochondrial ATP hydrolysis catalyzed by the F0F1-ATPase and we found that this activity increases significantly in patients with probable AD as compared to the control subjects. However, the transmembrane pH gradient driven by ATP hydrolysis was lower in

AD samples as compared to the controls (0.5 ± 0.1 pH units). This suggests a functional alteration of the FOF1-ATPase [45].

The fluidity of plasma membrane of erythrocytes were not modified significantly in samples of Mexican AD patients compared to healthy controls, regardless of increased lipid oxidation in erythrocytes AD patients. These data were similar to the previously reported [52] This suggests that inner mitochondrial membranes are more sensitive to oxidative stress than erythrocytes. it has been reported an increase in fluidity in whole membranes from platelets of AD patients [53]. This increase is due to a functionally abnormal membrane compartment resembling endoplasmic reticulum [54]. It is worth noting that platelets contain a few mitochondria, therefore, the contribution of mitochondrial membranes to the whole cell membranes is minimal [55]. Additionally, we found a significant decrease of membrane fluidity in hippocampal neurons from AD patients compared with membranes from elderly non demented controls. Lower membrane fluidity in AD patients was correlated with abnormal APP processing and cognitive decline [56].

The human cytochrome c oxidase is the terminal enzyme complex of the respiratory chain; it is located in the inner mitochondrial membrane where it catalyzes the transfer of electrons from reduced cytochrome c to molecular oxygen. Mitochondrial cytochrome c oxidase (MTCO) is made up of 13 subunits; its catalytic core is made up from the protein products of the MTCO I, II, and III genes that are encoded in mitochondrial DNA. Diminished cytochrome c oxidase activity has been described in AD postmortem cerebral cortex [57-60] and platelets [61]. Kish et al. [62] reported a reduced level of this protein complex in AD brain. These data could suggest that brain cytochrome oxidase is kinetically abnormal; thus, this dysfunction must arise from a catalytic defect rather than an underproduction [61]. However, mutations of the mitochondrial genome are widely recognized as important causes of disease [63]. Analysis of mitochondrial cytochrome c oxidase II gene obtained from blood samples of Mexican patients with AD revealed that 4 nonrelated patients with probable AD harbored the polymorphism A8027G (three of them were diagnosed with LOAD, with familial history of the disease and one of them with EOAD. This polymorphism shows a frequency of 12% in the analyzed sample. Four patients with EOAD harbored only one of thefollowing point mutations: A8003C, T8082C, C8201T, andG7933A, respectively. The A8003C transversion converts a polar neutral asparagine residue to a basic histidine. The T8082C transition converts proline to a leucine. C8201T transition converts a nonpolar aromatic phenylalanine to a nonpolar leucine. G7603A transversion converts a basic arginine to a basic histidine. From the 33 patients that were enrolled for this study only 8 of them presented a nucleotide variation in MTCO II gene, representing the 24% of the total of the patients. Three of the eight patients (37.5%) showed nucleotide variation and were diagnosed with LOAD. While, five of the eight patients (62.5%) were EOAD [64].

6. Histopathology of EOAD

Definitive diagnosis of AD late/onset is based on examination of brain tissue obtained at autopsy. The histopathology of EOAD is a neurodegenerative process characterized by selective and progressive death of neuronal cells in specific brain areas, primarily in the neocortex and hippocampus, which is clinically reflected by a dementia state. The clinical picture of dementia AD is accompanied by a massive buildup of insoluble filaments having ß-folded conformation which define two main types of lesions: neuritic plaques (NP) and neurofibrillary tangles (NFT) (figures 6-8). The major protein component of the NP fibrils is the beta-amyloid peptide and the NFT, tau. In general, it should be noted that both the formation of fibrils ß amyloid as the PNs of NFT.

The NP are composed of two main components: a core of extracellular amyloid ß and an arrangement of nerve terminals degenerate, uniquely shaped, dystrophic neurites, which may be intracellular or extracellular nature depending on their state of degeneration. These neurites surround the core board. Characteristically NP in EOAD are surrounded by numerous glial cells which, in encapsulate way. NP density correlates with the degree of the EOAD. In the case of Alzheimer's, as well as in healthy older adults can be found in the brain amyloid deposits without neuritic ß component. Unlike NP, this type of injury, called senile plaque, not correlated with EA. These findings have suggested that senile plaques are a risk factor for the development of the disease, that is, its presence is necessary but not sufficient for the onset.

The number of NFT observed in post-mortem histology of Alzheimer's cases correlate with the severity and duration of dementia. The NFT can be of two types: intracellular and extracellular depending if they are within the neuron or in the extracellular space with the death of the same. There are ways to evolve as the NFT changes from one state to another. It is clear that the dystrophic neurites are also part of the fibrillary degeneration of neuronal cells. Neurites are formed from the accumulation of abnormal filaments at the terminals of the cell axons and dendrites.

In OEAD the evolution of neurofibrillary formation in the hippocampus is very fast, the NFT appear in greater numbers in the transition zone (trans-enthorinal) and its adjacent layer II of the enthorinal cortex, which are located in the parahippocampal, temporal lobe. This information is key to understanding the pathophysiology of EOAD and its rapid development as well as its clinical correlation, since neuronal cells of layer II (enthorinal) on cortex relay zone where axons of associative neocortical areas arrive. The axons from layer II reach the hippocampus through a defined path via piercing call, and then synapse hippocampal pyramidal neuron. Once the information is processed, hippocampal axons synapse with output layer IV of the entorhinal cortex and hence the information to the entire neocortex is shipped. In other words the synaptic connections of the neocortex and the hippocampus is limited to the entorhinal cortex. In EOAD, to be destroyed these two layers also very fast; "off"... these two important areas of the brain, concomitant destruction of the hippocampus creates a complete disconnect with the associative areas of the neocortex

In Los Altos de Jalisco (Mexican region), there are many affected, even compare this (region) with others in the country, and in the world (the epidemiological analysis) exhibited a high prevalence. In autopsies members of these families show the basics of pathological diagnosis: a) neuritic plaques; b) neurofibrillary tangles; c) granulo-vacuolar degeneration; d) congophilic degeneration and Hirano body´s (these also observed in others pathologies).

The autopsy of a member family (3 affected) exhibited the typical diagnostic markers mentioned above; even using routine stains (H/E). Figure 6 exhibited degeneration and neuronal death (arrows); in the center of picture you can see the arrow labeled occupy the space surrounded by tangles neuron and glia.

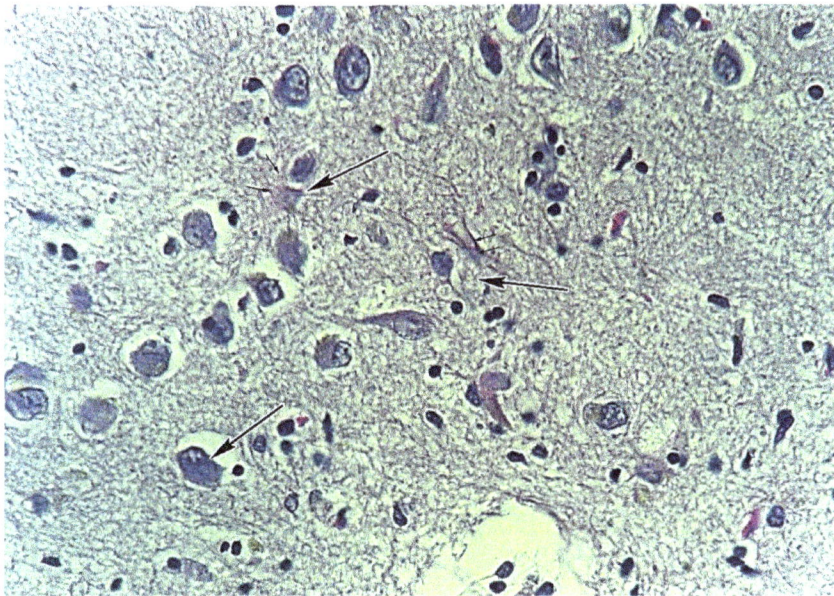

Figure 6. Exhibited the typical image of a neuritic plaques surrounded of gliosis (arrows).

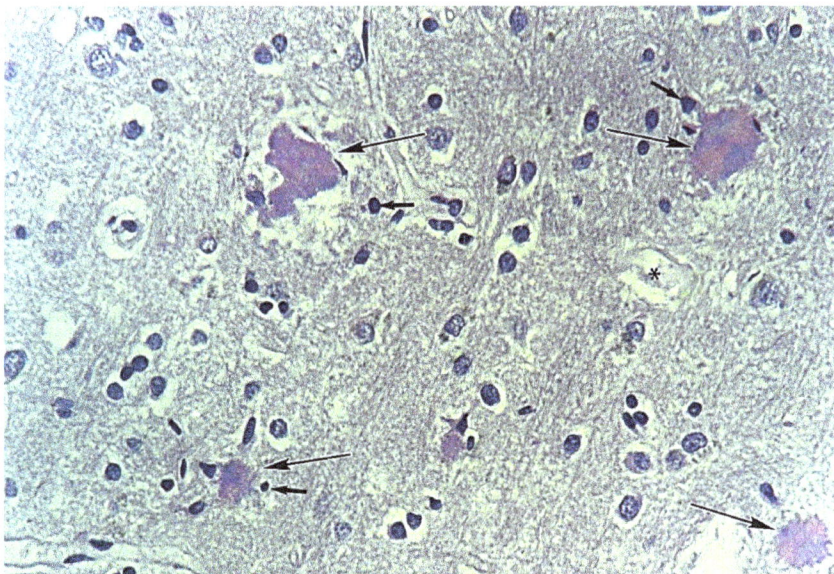

Figure 7. Exhibited in the center (arrows) a neuritic plaque, and marked with asterisks neurons showing intra/extra cellular tangles.

Neuritic plaques in EOAD are more complex; they consist of extracellular insoluble deposits formed by various compounds, the most abundant Aβ protein. This protein, as discussed above, is derived by proteolytic processing of a larger protein APP. The plates can be described as diffuse or classical. Diffuse are added amorphous Aβ are not associated with dystrophic neurites or abnormal neurons. Neuritic plaques are composed classical extracellular insoluble deposits formed by various compounds, the most abundant is the Aβ protein. This protein, as discussed above, is derived by proteolytic processing attic of a larger protein APP. The plates can be described as diffuse or classical. Diffuse are added amorphous Aβ, and are not associated with dystrophic neurites or abnormal neurons. Classical neuritic plaques contain fibrillar aggregates of dense insoluble Aβ surrounded dystrophic neurites, astrocytes and activated microglia assets which are associated with neuronal degeneration and loss. Containing dense fibrillar aggregates of amyloid β insoluble surrounded dystrophic neurites, astrocytes and activated microglia assets which are associated with neuronal degeneration and loss. In the vessels of the hippocampus and cortex, the existence of numerous neuritic plaques is observed. Neuritic plaques consist of clusters of axons degenerate dendritic spines and with a core containing extracellular linear filaments formed by the β-amyloid peptide. Amyloid deposits in senile plaques and in blood vessels of the cerebral cortex amyloid β fragment, whose amino acid sequence provided the basis for cloning the gene expressing the β amyloid was found. This gene encodes the APP protein, fragments that originates from proteolysis from 38 to 42 amino acids, the Aβ. In families with early disease has come to identify a place on the long arm of chromosome 21; duplicated in Down syndrome region near the gene encoding APP.

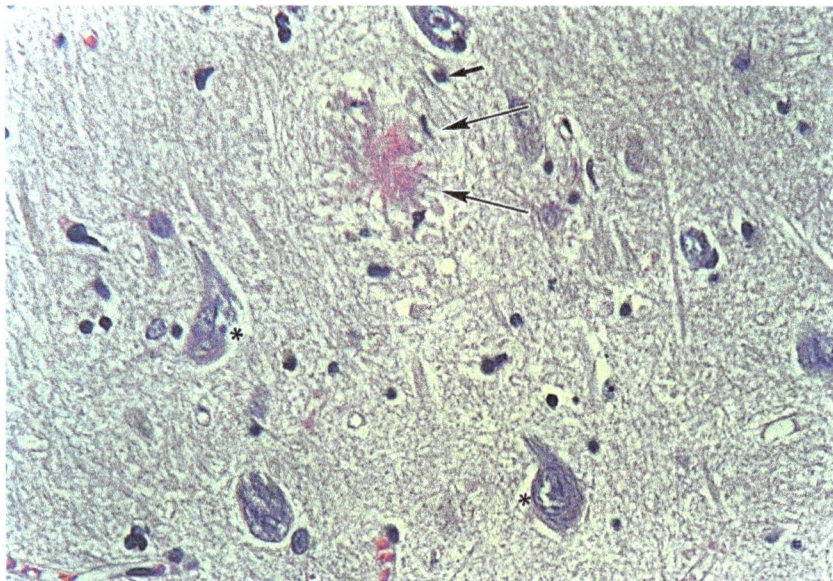

7. Neurofibrillary tangles in EOAD

Constitute one of the main lesions associated with the disease, and its presence is essential for diagnosis, Consist of abnormal fibrous inclusions in the perinuclear cytoplasm of neurons. The bulk density of neurofibrillary tangles in EOAD cases found in the neurons of the entorhinal cortex and CA1 region of the hippocampus and subiculum (layers III, V and VI of the neocortex). Several studies have shown a correlation between the load of neurofibrillary tangles and the degree of cognitive impairment, which has been correlated to these lesions have a direct effect on neuronal function. Despite being one of the cardinal lesions of AD is not pathognomonic of it. You can find (in addition to normal people) in other diseases such as: posttraumatic and pugilistic dementia or parkinsonism-dementia complex.

Finally the figure 9 exhibited the typical image of the granulo-vacuolar degeneration (arrows), and we appreciate the fine neuropil granulation, and fuzzy presence of tangles.

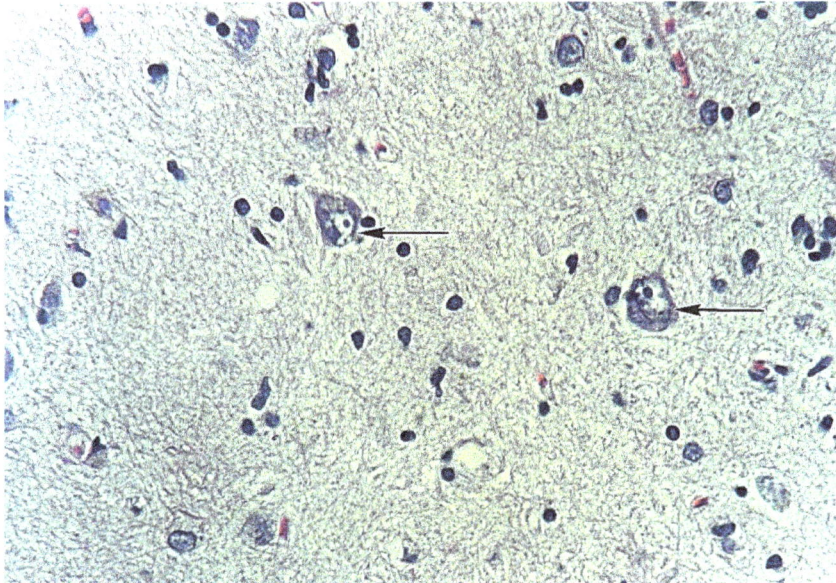

8. Granulovacuolar Degeneration in EOAD

Consists of an alteration of neurons in which the presence is observed in the cytoplasm of clustered small vacuoles, each of which contains a basophil granule inside, we observed this degeneration in all the hippocampus (also the enthorinal area). This granule appears to consist of several different proteins, such as neurofilament, tubulin, tau and ubiquitin among others. Little is known about the nature and significance of these alterations. Although you can find in elderly otherwise healthy brains, their presence in large numbers at the junction between the CA1 and CA2 regions of the hippocampus is strongly associated with AD.

Today it is a challenge the diagnosis of Alzheimer's... More interdisciplinary research is needed

Acknowledgements

Dr Raúl Mena-López (*in memoriam*)

Author details

Genaro Gabriel Ortiz[1*], Fermín P. Pacheco-Moisés[2], Erika D. González-Renovato[1],
Luis Figuera[3], Miguel A. Macías-Islas[4], Mario Mireles-Ramírez[5], L. Javier Flores-Alvarado[4],
Angélica Sánchez-López[1], Dhea G. Nuño-Penilla[1], Irma E. Velázquez- Brizuela[4],
Juan P. Sánchez-Luna[1] and Alfredo Célis de la Rosa[4]

*Address all correspondence to: genarogabriel@yahoo.com

1 División de Neurociencias. Centro de Investigación Biomédica de Occidente (CIBO), Instituto Mexicano del Seguro Social (IMSS). Guadalajara, Jalisco, México

2 Departamento de Química, Centro Universitario de Ciencias Exactas e Ingenierías. Universidad de Guadalajara. Guadalajara, Jalisco, México

3 División de Genética. Centro de Investigación Biomédica de Occidente, Instituto Mexicano del Seguro Social. Guadalajara, Jalisco, México

4 Centro Universitario de Ciencias de la Salud. Universidad de Guadalajara. Guadalajara, Guadalajara, Jalisco, México

5 Departamento de Neurología. Unidad Médica de Alta Especialidad (UMAE)- Hospital de Especialidades; Centro Médico Nacional de Occidente. Instituto Mexicano del Seguro Social (IMSS). Guadalajara, Jalisco, México

References

[1] Goedert M, Spillantini MG. (2006), A century of Alzheimer's disease. Science. 2006; 314:777-781.

[2] Goeder t M, Klug A, Crowther RA. Tau protein, the paired helical filament and Alzheimer's disease. Journal of Alzheimer's Disease. 2006; 9:195-207.

[3] Gong C-X, Liu F, Grundke-Iqbal I, Iqbal K. Dysregulation of protein phosphorylation/dephosphorylation in Alzheimer's disease: a therapeutic target. Journal of Biomedicine & Biotechnology. 2006;(article ID 31825):1-11.

[4] Zhou L-X, Zeng Z-Y, Du J-T, Zhao Y-F, Li Y-M. (2006), The self-assembly ability of the first microtubule-binding repeat from tau and its modulation by phosphorylation. Biochemical & Biophysical Research Communication. 2006; 348:637-642.

[5] Cruts, M. (2009). Alzheimer Disease & Frontotemporal Dementia Mutation Database. http://www.molgen.ua.ac.be/ADMutations/

[6] Farrall AJ, Wardlaw JM. Blood-brain barrier: ageing and microvascular disease systematic review and meta-analysis. Neurobiol Aging. 2009; 30: 337–52.

[7] Popescu BO, Toescu EC, Popescu LM. Blood-brain barrier alterations in ageing and dementia. J Neurol Sci. 2009; 283: 99–106.

[8] Cacabelos R, Fernandez-Novoa L, Lombardi V, Kubota Y, Takeda M. Molecular genetics of Alzheimer's disease and aging. Methods Find Exp Clin Pharmacol 27, Suppl A: 1–573, 2005.

[9] Turner RS. Alzheimer's Disease. Seminars in Neurology. 2006; 26(5):499-506.

[10] Price JL, Morris JC. Tangles and plaques in nondemented aging and "preclinical" Alzheimer's disease. Ann Neurol 1999;45:358-368.

[11] Delabio R, Rasmussen L, Mizumoto I, Viani GA, Chen E, Villares J, Costa IB, Turecki G, Linde SA, Smith MC, Payão SL.PSEN1 and PSEN2 Gene Expression in Alzheimer's Disease Brain: A New Approach. J Alzheimers Dis. 2014 Jan 1;42(3):757-60.

[12] Kim DH, Yeo SH, Park JM, Choi JY, Lee TH, Park SY, Ock MS, Eo J, Kim HS, Cha HJ.Gene. 2014 Jul 25;545(2):185-93.

[13] Jiao B, Tang B, Liu X, Xu J, Wang Y, Zhou L, Zhang F, Yan X, Zhou Y, Shen L. Mutational analysis in early-onset familial Alzheimer's disease in Mainland China. Neurobiol Aging. 2014 Aug;35(8):1957.e1-6. doi: 10.1016/j.neurobiolaging.2014.02.014.

[14] Wu L, Rosa-Neto P, Hsiung GY, Sadovnick AD, Masellis M, Black SE, Jia J, Gauthier S. Early-onset familial Alzheimer's disease (EOFAD). Can J Neurol Sci. 2012 Jul;39(4): 436-45.

[15] Kim DH, Yeo SH, Park JM, Choi JY, Lee TH, Park SY, Ock MS, Eo J, Kim HS, Cha HJGenetic markers for diagnosis and pathogenesis of Alzheimer's disease. Gene. 2014 Jul 25;545(2):185-93. doi: 10.1016/j.gene.2014.05.031.

[16] Pilotto A, Padovani A, Borroni B. Clinical, biological, and imaging features of monogenic Alzheimer's Disease. Biomed Res Int. 2013;2013:689591.

[17] El Kadmiri N, Hamzi K, El Moutawakil B, Slassi I, Nadifi S. Genetic aspects of Alzheimer's disease. Pathol Biol (Paris). 2013 Dec;61(6):228-38.

[18] Michikawa M. Role of apolipoprotein E in the molecular pathomechanism of Alzheimer disease. Nihon Shinkei Seishin Yakurigaku Zasshi. 2014 Feb;34(1):5-9. Review. Japanese. PMID: 2506926

[19] Nicolas M, Hassan BA. Amyloid precursor protein and neural development. Development. 2014 Jul;141(13):2543-8. doi: 10.1242/dev.108712.

[20] Jiang T, Yu JT, Tian Y, Tan L. Epidemiology and etiology of Alzheimer's disease: from genetic to non-genetic factors. Curr Alzheimer Res. 2013 Oct;10(8):852-67.

[21] Rahman B, Meiser B, Sachdev P, Barlow-Stewart K, Otlowski M, Zilliacus E, Schofield P. To know or not to know: an update of the literature on the psychological and

behavioral impact of genetic testing for Alzheimer disease risk. Genet Test Mol Biomarkers. 2012 Aug;16(8):935-42.

[22] Wain KE, Uhlmann WR, Heidebrink J, Roberts JS. Living at risk: the sibling's perspective of early-onset Alzheimer's disease. J Genet Couns. 2009 Jun;18(3):239-51.

[23] Ringman JM, C, Diaz-Olavarrieta Y, Rodriguez M, Chavez F, Paz, J, Murrell M,Macias-Islas M, Hil Kawas. Female preclinical presenilin-1 mutation carriers unaware of their genetic status have higher levels of depression than their non-mutation carrying kin. J Neurol Neurosurg Psychiatry 2004; 75 :500–502. doi: 10.1136/jnnp.2002.005025

[24] Ringman JM, Diaz-Olavarrieta,Y, Rodriguez, Chavez M,. Fairbanks F, Paz A, Varpetian HC, Maldonado M,. Macias-Islas M, J. Murrell JB, Ghetti l, Kawas C. Neuropsychological function in nondemented carriers of presenilin-1 mutations. NEUROLOGY 2005;65:552–558

[25] Ringman JM, Rodriguez Y, Diaz-Olavarrieta C, Michael T, Fairbanks L, Paz F, Varpetian, Chaparro H, Macias-Islas M, Murrell J, Bernardino Ghetti B, Kawas C. Performance on MMSE sub-items and education level in presenilin-1mutation carriers without dementia International Psychogeriatric Association 2006;2-10 doi:10.1017/S10416102060037

[26] Murrell J, Ghetti B, Cochran E, Macias-Islas M, Medina L, Varpetian A, Jeffrey L. Cummings LJ, Mario, Mendez MF, Claudia Kawas C, Helena Chui, Ringman JM. The A431E mutation in PSEN1 causing Familial Alzheimer's Disease originating in Jalisco State, Mexico: an additional fifteen families. Neurogenetics DOI 10.1007/s10048-006-0053-1

[27] Corder EH. Gene dose of apolipoprotein E type 4 allele and the risk of Alzheimer's disease in late onset families. Science, 1993; 261(5123): 921-3.

[28] Fagan AM. Unique lipoproteins secreted by primary astrocytes from wild type, apoE (-/-), and human apoE transgenic mice. J Biol Chem. 1999; 274(42): 30001-7.

[29] Gong JS. Apolipoprotein E (apoE) isoform-dependent lipid release from astrocytes prepared from human-apoE3- and apoE4-knock-in mice. J Biol Chem, 2002; 31: 31.

[30] Vance JE, Hayashi H. Formation and function of apolipoprotein E-containing lipoproteins in the nervous system. Biochim Biophys Acta. 2010; 1801(8): 806-18.

[31] Boyles JK. A role for apolipoprotein E, apolipoprotein A-I, and low density lipoprotein receptors in cholesterol transport during regeneration and remyelination of the rat sciatic nerve. J. Clin. Invest., 1989; 83: 1015-1031.

[32] Gong JS. Novel action of apolipoprotein E (ApoE): ApoE isoform specifically inhibits lipid-particle-mediated cholesterol release from neurons. Mol Neurodegener, 2007; 2: 9.LaDu MJ. Association of human, rat, and rabbit apolipoprotein E with beta amyloid. J Neurosci Res. 1997;. 49(1): 9-18.

[33] Golabek AA, Kida, E, Walus M, Perez C, Wisniewski, T, Soto C. Sodium dodecyl sulfate-resistant complexes of Alzheimer's amyloid beta-peptide with the N-terminal, receptor binding domain of apolipoprotein E. Biophys J. 2000; 79, 1008-1015.

[34] Tamamizu-Kato S, Cohen JK, Drake CB, Kosaraju MG, Drury J, Narayanaswami V. Interaction with Amyloid beta Peptide Compromises the Lipid Binding Function of Apolipoprotein E. Biochemistry; 2008.

[35] Consensus report of the Working Group on: "Molecular and Biochemical Markers of Alzheimer's Disease". The Ronald and Nancy Reagan Research Institute of the Alzheimer's Association and the National Institute on Aging Working Group. Neurobiol Aging. 1998; 19:109-116.

[36] Price JL and Morris JC. Tangles and plaques in nondemented aging and "preclinical" Alzheimer's disease. Ann Neurol 1999;45:358-368.

[37] Neuropathology Group. Medical Research Council Cognitive Function and Aging Study. Pathological correlates of late-onset dementia in a multicentre, community-based population in England and Wales. Neuropathology Group of the Medical Research Council Cognitive Function and Ageing Study (MRC CFAS). Lancet. 2001; 357:169-175.

[38] Herukka S-K, Hallikainen M, Soininen H, Pirttilä T. CSF Aβ42 and Tau or phosphorylated Tau and prediction of progressive mild cognitive impairment. Neurology. 2005; 64, 1294-1297

[39] Saez-Valero J, Barquero MS, Marcos A, McLean GA, Small DH. Altered glycosylation of acetylcholinesterase in lumbar cerebrospinal fluid of patients with Alzheimer's disease. J Neurol Neurosurg Psychiatry. 2000; 69:664-667.

[40] Bonelli RM, Aschoff A, Niederwieser G, Heuberger C, Jirikowski G. Cerebrospinal fluid tissue transglutaminase as a biochemical marker for Alzheimer's disease. Neurobiol Dis 2002;11:106-110.

[41] Leoni V, Shafaati M, Salomon A, Kivipelto M, Bjorkhem I, Wahlund LO. Are the CSF levels of 24S-hydroxycholesterol a sensitive biomarker for mild cognitive impairment?. Neurosci Lett. 2006; 397:83-87.

[42] Montine TJ, Kaye JA, Montine KS, McFarland L, Morrow JD, Quinn JF. Cerebrospinal fluid Aβ42, tau and F2-isoprostane concentrations in patients with Alzheimer's disease, other dementias, and in age.matched controls. Arch Pathol Lab Med. 2001;125:510-512.

[43] Simonsen AH, McGuire J, Hansson O, Zetterberg H, Podust VN, Davies HA, et al. Novel panel of Cerebrospinal fluid biomarkers for the prediction of progression to Alzheimer dementia in patients with mild cognitive impairment. Arch Neurol. 2007; 64:366-370.

[44] Blennow K. Cerebrospinal fluid protein biomarkers for Alzheimer's disease. Neu-roRx. 2004; 1:213-225-

[45] Martínez-Cano, E., Pacheco-Moisés, F.P., Ortiz, G.G., Macías-Islas, M.A., Sánchez-Nieto, S., and Rosales-Corral, S.A. 2004, Rev. Neurol., 39, 1

[46] Sánchez-González, V.J., Ortiz, G.G., Gallegos-Arreola, P., Macías-Islas, M.A., et al., Altered β-amyloid precursor protein isoforms in Mexican Alzheimer's Disease patients J.J. 2006, Dis. Markers, 22, 119.

[47] Mecocci, P., Cherubinia, A., Flint Beal, M. et al., 1996, Neurosc Lett., 207,129, 132.

[48] Borroni B., F. Colciaghi, C. Caltagirone et al., Platelet amyloid precursor protein abnormalities in Mild Cognitive Impairment predict conversion to dementia of Alzhemier type, Arch Neurol 60 (2003), 1740–1744.

[49] Mayeux R., A. Saunders, S. Shea et al., Utility of the apolipoprotein E genotype in the diagnosis of Alzheimer's disease, NEJM 338 (1998), 506–511.

[50] Ortiz G.G., F. Pacheco-Moises, M. El Hafidi, A. Jimenez-Delgado, M.A. Macias-Islas,S.A. et al. Detection of membrane fluidity in submitochondrial particles of platelets and erythrocyte membranes from Mexican patients with Alzheimer disease by intramolecular excimer formation of 1,3 dipyrenylpropane. Dis Markers 2008:(24) 151-156.

[51] Bonilla E, K. Tanji, M. Hirano, T.H. Vu, S. DiMauro, E.A. Schon, Mitochondrial involvement in Alzheimer's disease. Biochim Biophys Acta 1999:(1410) 171-182.

[52] Hajimohammadreza I, Brammer MJ, Eagger S, Burns A, Levy R. Platelet and erythrocyte membrane changes in Alzheimer's disease. Biochim Biophys Acta. 1990; (1025): 208-214.

[53] Zubenko GS, Kopp U, Seto T, Firestone LL. Platelet membrane fluidity individuals at risk for Alzheimer's disease: a comparison of results from fluorescence spectroscopy and electron spin resonance spectroscopy. Psychopharmacology. 1999; (145): 175-180.

[54] Zubenko GS, Malinakova I, Chojnacki B. Proliferation of internal membranes in platelets from patients with Alzheimer's disease.. J Neuropathol Exp Neurol. 1987; (46): 407-418.

[55] Fukami MH, Salganicoff L. Isolation and properties of human platelet mitochondria. Blood. 1973; (42): 913-918.

[56] Zainaghi IA, Forlenza OV, Gattaz WF. Abnormal APP processing in platelets of patients with Alzheimer's disease: correlations with membrane fluidity and cognitive decline. Psychopharmacology (Berl). 2007; (192): 547-553.

[57] Kish SJ, Bergeron C, Rajput A. Brain cytochrome oxidase in Alzheimer's disease. Journal of Neurochemistry. 1992; 59 (2):. 776–779.

[58] Mutisya EM, Bowling AC, Beal MF. Cortical cytochrome oxidase activity is reduced in Alzheimer's disease. Journal of Neurochemistry. 1994; 63(6):.2179–2184.

[59] Parker WD Jr, Parks J, Filley CM, Kleinschmidt BK. Electron transport chain defects in Alzheimer's disease brain. Neurology. 1994; 44(6): 1090–1096.

[60] Valla J, Berndt JD, Lima FG. Energy hypometabolism in posterior cingulate cortex of Alzheimer's patients: superficial laminar cytochrome oxidase associated with disease duration. Journal of Neuroscience. 2001; 21(13): 4923–4930.

[61] Cardoso SM, Proenca MT, Santos S, Santana I, Oliveira CR. Cytochrome c oxidase is decreased in Alzheimer's disease platelets. Neurobiology of Aging. 2004; 25(1): 105–110.

[62] Kish S. J., C. Bergeron, A. Rajput et al., "Brain cytochrome oxidase in Alzheimer's disease," Journal of Neurochemistry, vol. 59, no. 2, pp. 776–779, 1992.

[63] Hirano M, A. Shtilbans, R. Mayeux et al., "Apparent mtDNA heteroplasmy in Alzheimer's disease patients and in normals due to PCR amplification of nucleus-embedded mtDNA pseudogenes," Proceedings of the National Academy of Sciences of the United States of America, vol. 94, no. 26, pp. 14894–14899, 1997

[64] Loera-Castañeda V, Lucila Sandoval-Ramírez, Fermín Paul PachecoMoisés, Miguel Ángel Macías-Islas et al. Novel Point Mutations and A8027G Polymorphism in Mitochondrial-DNA-Encoded Cytochrome c Oxidase II Gene in Mexican Patients with Probable Alzheimer Disease. International Journal of Alzheimer's Disease Volume 2014, Article ID 794530, 5 pages

5

The Cascade of Oxidative Stress and Tau Protein Autophagic Dysfunction in Alzheimer's Disease

Zhenzhen Liu, Peifu Li, Jiannan Wu, Yi Wang, Ping Li, Xinxin Hou, Qingling Zhang, Nannan Wei, Zhiquan Zhao, Huimin Liang and Jianshe Wei

Additional information is available at the end of the chapter

1. Introduction

Alzheimer's disease (AD) is the most common form of dementia in the elderly and a chronic neurodegenerative disease characterized by widespread degeneration of neurons. An estimated 37 million people worldwide currently have AD, which is estimated to increase to 65.7 million by 2030 and 115.4 million by 2050 [1]. It is a growing health concern in society because patients suffer from progressive functional impairments, emotional distress, loss of independence, and behavioral deficits. AD is characterized by the presence of two types of neuropathological hallmarks: senile plaques (SPs) and intracellular neurofibrillary tangles (NFTs). SPs predominantly consist of extracellular amyloid β-peptide (Aβ) deposits. NFTs are formed by intraneuronal aggregation of hyperphosphorylated tau. The amyloid cascade hypothesis theory proposes a dysregulation of amyloid precursor protein processing. This event leads to AD pathogenesis, which involves the aggregation of Aβ (particularly Aβ42), neuritic plaque formation, and consequently the formation of NFTs followed by the disruption of synaptic connections, neuronal death, and cognitive deficits (dementia) [2]. Increasing evidence suggests that Aβ oligomers may be the primary cause of AD because they have a greater correlation with dementia than insoluble Aβ42. Aβ also plays a crucial role in inducing neuronal oxidative stress [3]. Aβ-mediated mitochondrial oxidative stress causes hyperphosphorylation of tau in AD brains [4, 5]. Mounting evidence clearly links tau to neurodegeneration, indicating that tau hyperphosphorylation may be the necessary link in neural dysfunction and death. However, whether autophagic dysfunction is involved in neuronal death during this event still remains unknown. Recent studies have indicated the importance of defective autophagy in the pathogenesis of aging and neurodegenerative diseases, especially in AD. Autophagy may increase the formation of autophagosome in AD, and autophagic dysfunction may induce the pathogenesis of AD, particularly at the late stage of AD [6]. However, the relationship between oxidative stress, tau protein hyperphosphorylation, autophagic dysfunction and neuronal cells death in AD remains elusive. In this review, we summarize the latest progress in research focused on oxidative stress, tau hyperphosphorylation, and autophagic dysfunction, and their relationship with AD.

2. Oxidative stress in AD

Oxidative stress appears to be one of the earliest events and a major determinant of the pathogenesis and progression in AD. In experimental models and human brain studies of AD, oxidative stress has also been shown to play an important role in neuronal degeneration [7]. Several risk factors for AD may cause or promote oxidative damage, such as advanced age, apolipoprotein E (APOE) ε4 alleles [8], medical risk factors, environmental and lifestyle-related risk factors and so on. Generally, oxidative stress is caused by the imbalance between reactive oxygen species (ROS) (O^{2-}, H_2O_2 and OH), which associated with both the chronic formation of ROS derived from the mitochondrial electron transport chain and the acute and high output formation of ROS derived from nicotinamide adenine dinucleotide phosphate (NADPH) oxidase, and the breakdown of chemically reactive species, by reducing agents and antioxidant enzymes, such as superoxide dismutase (SOD). This disequilibrium may result from disease, stressors, or environmental factors. High ROS levels lead to the accumulation of oxidized proteins, lipids, and nucleic acids due to mitochondrial dysfunction, increased metal levels, inflammation, and Aβ peptides, thereby directly impairing cellular function if not be removed or neutralized [9]. Oxidative damage to cellular components is likely to result in the alteration of membrane properties, such as fluidity, ion transport, enzyme activities, protein cross-linking, and eventually cell death.

Structurally and functionally damaged mitochondria are more proficient at producing ROS [10]. Mitochondrial dysfunction may be an initial trigger for enhanced Aβ production during the aging process [11].Oxidative stress can promote Aβ deposition, tau hyperphosphorylation, and the subsequent loss of synapses and neurons in the development of AD. Several studies suggest that ROS are involved in Aβ fibrillization and NFT formation in AD and increases with Aβ and NFT pathology in AD. Both soluble and fibrillar Aβ may further accelerate oxidative stress, as well as mitochondrial dysfunction [12-14]. The transgenic (Tg) Thy1-APP751 (SL) mouse model of AD shows increased proteolytic cleavage of APP, increased production of Aβ, and impaired Cu/Zn-SOD activity [15]. Furthermore, oxidative stress is considered as a primary factor of NFT formation in AD. However, the relationship between oxidative stress and tau hyperphosphorylation remains unclear. Okadaic acid is used as a research model to induce tau phosphorylation and neuronal death in AD. Oxidative stress combined with Okadaic acid results in tau hyperphosphorylation [16], and mitochondrial SOD_2 deficiency also increases the levels of Ser396 phosphorylated tau in the Tg2576 mouse model of AD [4].

3. Tau protein in AD

3.1. Tau protein physiology and pathology

Tau protein (known as neuronal microtubule associated protein tau) plays a large role in the outgrowth of neuronal processes and the development of neuronal polarity. Tau protein in the central nervous system is predominantly expressed in neurons [17, 18], with its main function to promote microtubule assembly, stabilize microtubules, affect the dynamics of microtubules in neurons [19, 20], and inhibit apoptosis [21], particularly in axons [22, 23]. However, recent reports suggest that excess intracellular tau is released into the extracellular culture medium via membrane vesicles [24]. In the adult human brain, tau consists of six isoforms, and the tau gene contains 15 exons. The isoforms are generated by alternative splicing of exons 2, 3, and 10. Depending on the alternative splicing of exon 10, tau isoforms are termed 4R (with exon 10) or 3R (without exon 10). N-terminal exon (tau 1N), two N-terminal exons (tau 2N), or no N-terminal exons (tau 0N) at the N-terminal inserts mainly depend on the inclusion of exon 2, exon 2 and 3, or the exclusion of both. Biochemical analysis of postmortem AD brains indicate that 4R-tau is more abundant than 3R in isolated NFTs [25].

Tau protein normally stabilizes axonal microtubules in the cytoskeleton and plays a vital role in regulating the morphology of neurons. It has more than 30 phosphorylation sites. When tau is abnormally hyperphosphorylated, it destabilizes microtubules by decreasing the binding affinity of tau and resulting in its aggregation in NFTs. NFTs are composed of paired helical filaments (PHF) of abnormally hyperphosphorylated tau. The severity of dementia in AD was shown to correlate well with NFT load. In the transgenic mouse model, conditionally expressing the human tau P301L mutant, age-related NFTs develop, along with neuronal loss and behavioral impairment. After the suppression of transgenic tau, memory function recovered, and neuron numbers stabilized [26]. The pathogenesis of tau-mediated neurodegeneration is unclear but hyperphosphorylation, oligomerization, fibrillization, and propagation of tau pathology has been proposed as the likely pathological processes that induces the loss of function or gain of tau toxicity, which caused neurodegeneration [27]. Tau phosphorylation has been investigated at AD-related sites by using recombinant human tau phosphorylated by DNA damage-activated checkpoint kinase 1 (Chk1) and checkpoint kinase 2(Chk2) in vitro [28]. This study identified a total of 27 Ser/Thr residues as Chk1 or Chk2 target sites. Among these sites, 13 sites have been identified to be phosphorylated in AD brains [29]. The generation of a Tg mouse line overexpressing human tau 441 via V337M and R406W tau mutations has been shown to accelerate the phosphorylation of human tau, inducing tau pathology and cognitive deficits [30].

3.2. Tau protein kinases and phosphatase

Tau phosphorylation is mainly determined by a balance between the activation of various tau protein kinases and phosphatases, and its disruption results in the abnormal phosphorylation of tau, which is observed in AD. Each tau site is phosphorylated by one or more protein kinases. Tau kinases are grouped into three classes: (1) proline-directed protein kinases (PDPK) containing glycogen synthase kinase-3 (GSK3), cyclin-dependent protein kinase-5 (CDK5), and mitogen activated protein kinases (MAPK) (e.g. p38, Erk1/2 and JNK1/2/3); (2) non-PDPK, including tau-tubulin kinase 1/2 (e.g. casein kinase $1\alpha/1\delta/1\epsilon/2$), dual specificity tyrosine-phosphorylation-regulated kinase 1A/2, microtubule affinity regulating kinases, phosphorylase kinase, cAMP-dependent protein kinase A (PKA), PKB/Akt, protein kinase C, protein kinase N, and Ca2+/calmodulin-dependent protein kinase II (CaM kinase II); and (3) tyrosine protein kinases, including Src family kinase (SFK) members (e.g. Src, Lck, Syk, and Fyn), and c-Abelson kinase or Abl related gene kinase. Phosphatases are also usually classified into three classes according to their amino acids sequences, the structure of their catalytic site, and their sensitivity to inhibitors. These groups include: (1) phosphoprotein phosphatase (PPP), (2) metal-dependent protein phosphatase, and (3) protein tyrosine phosphatase (PTP).

GSK3 (particularly GSK3β) plays a key role in the pathogenesis of AD, contributing to Aβ production and Aβ-mediated neuronal death by phosphorylating tau in most serine and threonine residues and inducing hyperphosphorylation in paired helical filaments [31]. Inhibition of GSK3 prevents Aβ aggregation and tau hyperphosphorylation [32, 33]. The involvement of CDK5 in tau phosphorylation is shown by the increase in its enzymatic activity and the absence of MT-2 cells neurite retraction in the presence of roscovitine or CDK5 siRNA [34]. Therefore, CDK5 may be a key candidate target for therapeutic gene silencing [35]. p38 MAPK has been identified as one of the kinases involved in the regulation of tau phosphorylation. Thus, under pathological conditions this kinase is likely to play a role in the hyperphosphorylation of tau [36]. CDKs and casein kinase 1 (CK1) are involved in the aggregation of Aβ peptides (forming extracellular plaques) and hyperphosphorylation of tau (forming intracellular NFTs). The expression pattern of CKIδ (an isoform of CK1) plays an important role in tau aggregation in AD [37]. Ser214, Ser262, and Ser409 are major phosphorylation sites of tau that are affected by PKA [38]. In P19 cells stably expressing human tau441, CaM kinase II has been shown to be involved in retinoic acid (RA)-induced tau phosphorylation- mediated apoptosis [39].

Tau protein phosphatase PPP group includes protein phosphatase [PP]1, PP2A, PP2B and proteinphophatase-5 [PP5]. In vitro, Overexpression of PP5 resulted in dephosphorylation of tau at multiple phosphorylation sites [40] and protected neurons against apoptosis induced by Aβ [41]. In vivo, PP5 interacts with the regulatory subunit A of PP2A [42], and the enzymatic activity level of PP5 has been reduced by 20% in AD brains [40]. PP2A contributes to abnormally hyperphosphorylated tau protein, and is the most efficient phosphatase. The inhibition of PP2A significantly plays a role in tau hyperphosphorylation [43-45]. PP2A is regulated by endogenous inhibitor-1 of PP2A (I1PP2A) and inhibitor-2 of PP2A (I2PP2A) in mammalian tissues [46].

Recently inactivation the nuclear translocation signal (179KRK181-AAA) along with 168KR169-AA mutations of I2PP2A (mNLS-I2PP2A), it was translocated from nucleus to the cytoplasm. Cytoplasmic retention of I2PP2A physically interacted with PP2A and inhibited its activity, induced Alzheimer-like abnormal tau protein hyperphosphorylation by the direct interaction of I2 PP2A with PP2A and GSK-3β [47]. In AD brain, I2PP2A is also translocated from neuronal nucleus to cytoplasm, leading to the inhibition of PP2A and abnormal phosphorylation of tau. I2PP2A directly inhibits the activity of PP2A activity without affecting its expression [48]. Over activation of GSK-3β inhibits PP2A through up regulation of I2PP2A. GSK-3 activation significantly contributes to tau hyperphosphorylation by inhibiting PP2A via the up-regulation of I2PP2A [49]. These data indicate that up-regulation or down-regulation of the phosphorylation system or dephosphorylation system, respectively of tau protein may be implicated in tau pathologies.

3.3. Tau protein and oxidative stress

3.3.1. Tau protein hyperphosphorylation and oxidative stress

Oxidative stress is believed to be a prominent early event in the pathogenesis of AD, contributing to tau phosphorylation and the formation of neurofibrillary tangles. However, the relationship and underlying mechanisms between oxidative stress and tau hyperphosphorylation remains elusive. Fatty acid oxidative products provide a direct link between the mechanism of how oxidative stress induces the formation of NFTs in AD [50]. Chronic oxidative stress increases the levels of tau phosphorylation at paired helical filaments (PHF-1) epitope (serine 399/404) via the inhibition of glutathione synthesis with buthionine sulfoximine (BSO) in an vitro model of chronic oxidative stress [5]. In primary rat cortical neuronal cultures stimulated by the combination of the copper chelator, cuprizone, and oxidative stress (Fe^{2+}/H_2O_2), tau phosphorylation is significantly increased by the elevated activity of GSK-3 [51]. Furthermore, treatment of rat hippocampal cells and SHSY5Y human neuroblastoma cells with H_2O_2 at the early stages of oxidative stress exposure results in tau dephosphorylation at the Tau1 epitope by CDK5 via PP1 activation [52]. Several studies have suggested that oxidative stress is a causal factor in tau-induced neurodegeneration in Drosophila [53], and ROS generation is a key intracellular event that contributes to an induction of p38-MAPK activation and tau phosphorylation.

3.3.2. GSK3β, PP2A, and oxidative stress

Oxidative stress is likely to play a critical role in tau hyperphosphorylation, which is regulated by tau protein kinase activation and the suppression of phosphatase. Tau hyperphosphorylation may be induced by oxidative stress through the direct interaction with tau protein kinase and phosphatase, particularly GSK-3β and PP2A, respectively because they are predominant and play an important role.

The main site of ROS formation is mitochondrial complex I, inhibition of complex I induces a decrease in ATP levels and excessive production of ROS [54]. GSK-3β has been situated in the mitochondria and highly activated. Mitochondrial GSK3β activity controlled the mitochondrial complex I activity, promoted ROS production, and perturbed the mitochondrial morphology [55]. In contrast, GSK-3β activity is up-regulated under oxidative stress [56]. For example, in human embryonic kidney 293/Tau cells, H_2O_2 increases GSK-3β activity and tau is hyperphosphorylated at Ser396, Ser404, and Thr231. Mitochondrial superoxide activates the mitochondrial fraction of GSK-3α/β, resulting in the phosphorylation of the mitochondrial chaperone cyclophilin D [57]. This effect also provides a link between GSK-3β and oxidative stress.

Studies have also focused on the link between PP2A and oxidative stress. A recent report shows that rat cortical neurons treated with okadaic acid inhibits PP2A activity, resulting in an abnormal increase in mitochondrial ROS and mitochondrial fission [58]. Other findings reveal that ROS inhibits PP2A and PP5, leading to the activation of JNK and Erk1/2 pathways and subsequently caspase-dependent and -independent apoptosis of neuronal cells [59]. In vivo, after hypoxia exposure, the levels of activated form of GSK-3β was significantly increased in the hippocampus, while activated form of PP2A were significantly decreased [60]. Despite these studies, however, the relationship of GSK3 and PP2A with oxidative stress remains to be further investigated.

3.3.3. Antioxidants and the tau protein

In recent years, antioxidant therapy has received considerable attention as a promising approach for slowing the progression of AD. Research has focused on endogenous antioxidants (e.g. vitamins, coenzyme Q10, and melatonin) and the intake of dietary antioxidants, such as phenolic compounds that are flavonoids or non-flavonoids. This increased interest has thus strengthened the hypothesis that oxidative damage may be responsible for the cognitive and functional decline in AD patients. Melatonin is a free radical scavenger, clinical trial revealed that add-on prolonged-release melatonin had positive effects on cognitive functioning and sleep maintenance in AD patients compared with placebo [61]. The mechanism may be that melatonin can block tau hyperphosphorylation and microtubule disorganization under in vivo and vitro conditions [62-64] and also decreases the activity of GSK-3β [65]. Moreover, melatonin may be a potentially useful agent in the prevention and treatment of AD [66]. Demethoxycurcumin has been shown to inhibit the phosphorylation of both tau pS262 and pS396 in murine neuroblastoma N2A cells [67]. Curcumin reduced soluble tau and elevated heat shock proteins involved in tau clearance [68]. In addition, curcumin downregulated levels of phosphorylated tau, which may concerned with the upregulation in BAG2 levels in the neurons [69]. In addition, an association also exists between beta carotene and tau in AD patients [70]. Other experiments have shown that the active component of Ginkgo biloba, ginkgolide A, inhibits GSK3β and suppressed the phosphorylation level of tau [71]. Other antioxidants, such as Vitamins E and C [72, 73] and gossypin [74] are also reported to have a protective effect against neurotoxicity. These results have therefore led to further investigations of this compound as an antioxidant therapy strategy for AD.

4. Autophagy in AD

4.1. The Autophagic pathway

Autophagy is an essential lysosomal degradation pathway that turns over cytoplasmic constituents, including misfolded or aggregated proteins and damaged organelles, to facilitate the maintenance of cellular homeostasis. Autophagy is usually activated during nutrient deprivation and stress to enhance cellular survival, and its constitutive activity is recognized to control neuronal survival. Autophagic dysfunction has been reported to contribute to AD [75].

Autophagy includes macroautophagy, chaperone-mediated autophagy, and microautophagy. The most familiar of these types is macroautophagy, which is a process of cellular self-cannibalism in which portions of the cytoplasm are sequestered within double- or multimembraned vesicles (autophagosomes) and then delivered to lysosomes for bulk degradation. Autophagy is induced by two pathways in macroautophagy - mammalian target of rapamycin (mTOR)-dependent and -independent signaling pathways. mTOR is an important convergence point in the cell signaling pathway. mTOR kinase activity is modulated in response to various stimuli, such as trophic factors, mitogens, hormones, amino acids, cell energy status, and cellular stress. Rapamycin, as mTOR inhibitor, is a very important tool for autophagy [76, 77]. mTOR complex (mTORC) 1 is involved in autophagy and is the master regulator of cell growth enhancing the cellular biomass by up-regulating protein translation [78]. For cells to control cellular homoeostasis during growth, a close signaling interplay occurs between mTORC1 and two other protein kinases, AMP-activated protein kinase (AMPK) [79] and Unc51-like kinase (ULK1) [80]. Autophagy is inhibited by cytosolic p53 via the direct inhibition of AMPK [81]. mTORC1 controls autophagy by directly interacting with the ULK1, focal adhesion kinase family-interacting protein of 200 kDa (FIP200) and Atg13 complex [82]. Several mTOR-independent signals affect the autophagy pathway. When the level of free inositol and myoinositol-1,4,5- trisphosphate (IP3) decreases, autophagy is reduced [83]. Furthermore, lower levels of Bcl-2 lead to the release of more Beclin 1, thus forming the Beclin 1-PI3KCIII (class III phosphoinositide 3-kinase) complex to activate autophagy via the PI3K-AKT-mTOR pathway [84].

4.2. Autophagic dysfunction in AD pathology

A growing body of evidence suggests a link between AD and autophagy. Therefore, the pathological functions of autophagy may be a critical mediator of neurotoxicity [85]. Autophagy develops in AD brains because of the ineffective degradation of autophagosomes, which is controlled by many kinds of autophagy-related genes (Atg), including Atg1-Atg35. Atg8 (mammalian homolog is LC3) is an autophagosomal membrane protein and a marker of autophagosome formation [86]. Beclin-1 (the mammalian ortholog of yeast Atg6) plays a pivotal role in autophagy [87]. In an in vitro study of the pathogenesis of AD, Atg8/LC3 colocalizes with APP and LC3-positive autophagosomes are present [88]. Beclin-1 knockdown increases APP, APP-like proteins, APP-C-terminal fragments, and Aβ [89]. Atg5, Atg12, and LC3 are also associated with plaque, tangle pathologies, and neuronal death in AD [90]. Generally, autophagic vacuoles (AVs) are rare in the normal brain, but are increased in brains of AD patients. In the early stages of AD, the expression of lysosome-related component is significantly increased prior to the formation of plaques and NFTs, and autophagy is also induced at this stage, thus its activity is independent of extracellular Aβ deposition and NFT formation [91]. In the late stage of AD, AVs continue to accumulate in large numbers in dystrophic neurites. There are several causes for the dysfunction of autophagy in late-stage AD, including the enhanced processing of APP and Aβ degradation [92], and the toxic effect of high levels of intracellular Aβ on lysosomal function [93]. Inhibition of the AV-lysosome fusion is caused by impaired microtubule-associated retrograde transport, which in turn leads to increased accumulation of AV in dystrophic neurites. Lysosomal enzyme dysfunction may be associated with the accumulation of AVs [94, 95]. Autophagy plays an important role in the degradation of impaired mitochondria in AD. Dysfunction of the autophagy - lysosome system causes insufficient degradation of mitochondria [96]. Conversely, mitochondrial dysfunction may also impair this pathway [97].

4.3. Autophagy and the tau protein

4.3.1. Tau protein degradation via autophagy

A variety of forms of tau proteins have been shown to be degraded by the ubiquitin-proteasome system (UPS) and autophagy-lysosomal pathway (ALP). UPS may play an important role in the primary clearance of pathological tau. However, the importance of autophagy-mediated tau degradation, particularly at the late stage of NFT formation, is becoming more recognized. The autophagy-lysosomal pathway has the capacity to engulf protein aggregates and keep tau levels at a low level [98]. Autophagy is believed to be an evolutionarily conserved mechanism for intracellular degradation of proteins, such as Aβ and tau. mTOR in negatively regulating autophagy is an important convergence point in cell signaling. Increasing mTOR signaling facilitates tau pathology, and reducing this signaling ameliorates tau pathology [99]. Rapamycin has been reported to decrease tau phosphorylation at Ser214 in vitro, and reduce tau tangles and insoluble tau in vivo [100, 101]. In a tetracycline-inducible model [tau DeltaC (tauΔC)], tau is abnormally truncated at Asp ^{421}, and is cleared predominantly by macroautophagy and degraded significantly faster than full-length tau [102]. Autophagy activation suppresses tau aggregation and eliminates cytotoxicity [99]. Moreover, trehalose (an enhancer of autophagy) directly inhibits tau aggregation in primary neurons [103]. Under in vitro conditions, the accumulation of tau species is increased with the autophagic inhibitor, 3-methyladenine, and decreased with trehalose [104]. Overall, these results suggest that tau degradation involves autophagy, and this activity is beneficial for neurons to prevent the accumulation of protein aggregates.

4.3.2. Tau protein hyperphosphorylation leads to autophagic dysfunction

The physiological function of tau protein is well known to be associated with microtubule binding and assembly. Autophagosome transport mainly depends on the movement along microtubules in the autophagic pathway. However, the link between tau hyperphosphorylation and autophagic dysfunction is still under debate. Frontotemporal dementia and parkinsonism linked to chromosome 17 (FTDP-17) - mediated tau mutations can disrupt lysosomal function in transgenic mice expressing human Tau with four tubulin-binding repeats (increased by FTDP-17 splice donor mutations) and three FTDP-17 missense mutations: G272V, P301L, and R406W [105]. In Tg mice expressing mutant human (P301L) tau, axonal spheroids have been shown to contain tau-immunoreactive filaments and AVs [106]. A recent study has revealed that PP2A upregulation stimulates neuronal autophagy, thus providing link between PP2A downregulation, autophagy disruption, and protein aggregation [107]. Furthermore, autophagosomes have been shown to be increased in rat neurons treated with okadaic acid [108]. Altogether, tau is known to regulate the stability of microtubules, and tau hyperphosphorylation may result in the destabilization of neuronal microtubules, thus affecting the placement and function of mitochondria and lysosomes. Therefore, tau hyperphosphorylation is likely to play a critical role in the process of autophagic dysfunction.

4.3.3. Autophagic dysfunction induces tau protein aggregation

The autophagy-lysosomal pathway is well recognized to play an important role in the clearance of abnormally modified proteins in cells. The hyperphosphorylation of tau and NFT formation results in the disruption of the neuronal skeleton, thereby contributing to neuronal dysfunction, cell death, and eventually the symptoms of AD. Abnormal lysosomal proteases are found in brains of AD patients. Several studies have shown that dysfunction of the autophagy-lysosomal pathway contributes to the formation of tau oligomers and insoluble aggregates [109, 110]. Both phosphorylated tau and GSK3β significantly accumulate in Atg7 conditional knockout brains, although NFTs are absent [111]. Therefore, the ALP system plays a crucial role in the clearance of tau, and its accumulation may be due to autophagic dysfunction in cells.

5. Conclusion

Oxidative stress, as the one of the earliest events in AD, induces tau phosphorylation with protein phosphatase and kinase imbance. Tau protein hyperphosphorylation destabilizes

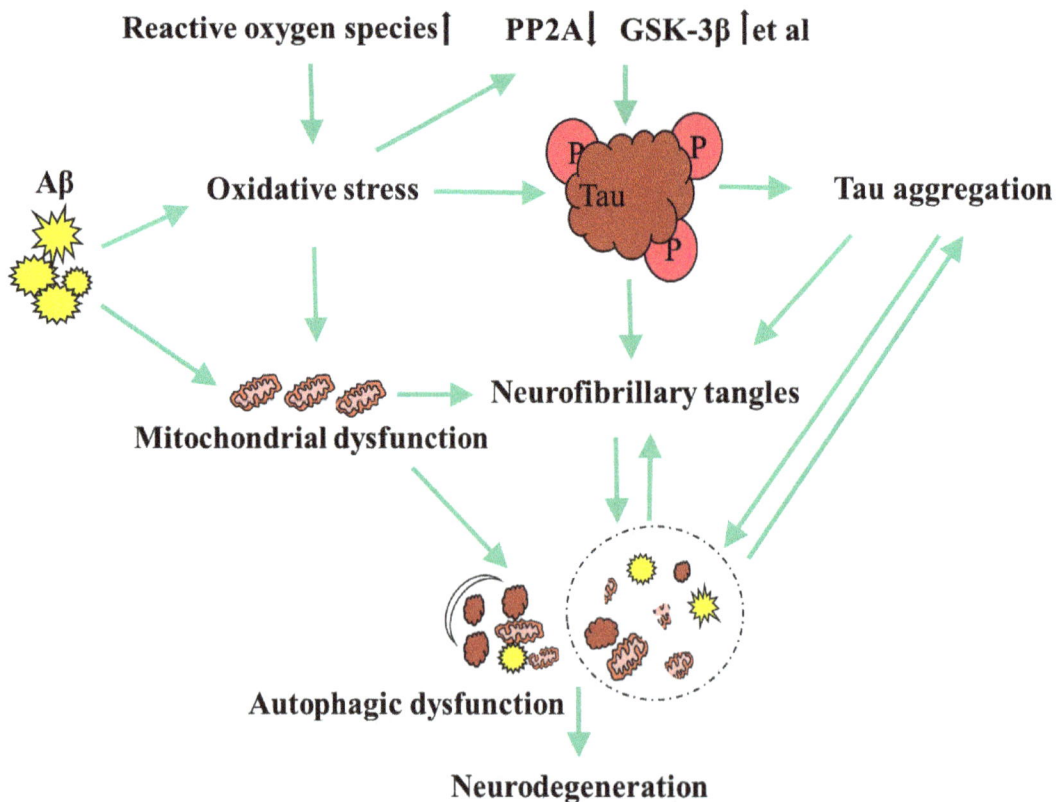

Figure 1. Tau protein NFTs formation and autophagic dysfunction in Alzheimer's disease. Aβ oligomers and ROS production intrigue oxidative stress and mitochondria dysfunction, which induce tau protein hyperphosphorylation and neurofibrillary tangles formation. These events converge to tau protein aggregation and autophagic dysfunction, then lead to neurodegeneration and cell death in AD.

microtubules by decreasing the binding affinity of tau, thereby resulting in the formation of NFTs in AD. Tau hyperphosphorylation may affect the autophagy- lysosomal pathway, and dysfunction of the ALP also promotes the accumulation of tau protein. These events initiate a series of cascades to induce neurodegeneration and cell death in AD (Figure 1). However, the relationships among oxidative stress, tau hyperphosphorylation and autophagic dysfunction and their accurate mechanisms on neurodegeneration in AD still require further research.

Acknowledgements

The work has been generously supported by grant from the National Natural Science Foundation of China (81271410 to JW). The authors thank all other authors making contributions to the studies cited in this manuscript and apologize to those who made similar contributions in work not being cited due to space limitation. The authors have no competing financial interests.

Author details

Zhenzhen Liu[1,2], Peifu Li[2], Jiannan Wu[1], Yi Wang[1], Ping Li[1], Xinxin Hou[2], Qingling Zhang[2], Nannan Wei[1], Zhiquan Zhao[1], Huimin Liang[1] and Jianshe Wei[1,2*]

*Address all correspondence to: jswei@henu.edu.cn

1 Laboratory of Brain Function and Molecular Neurodegeneration, Institute for Brain Science Research, School of Life Sciences, Henan University, Kaifeng, China

2 Institute of Neuroscience, Henan Polytechnic University, Jiaozuo, China

References

[1] Cumming T, Brodtmann A. Dementia and stroke: The present and future epidemic. International Journal of Stroke 2010; 5(6): 453-454.

[2] Lee HG, Zhu X, Nunomura A, Perry G, Smith MA. Amyloid beta: the alternate hypothesis. Current Alzheimer Research 2006; 3(1): 75-80.

[3] De Felice FG, Velasco PT, Lambert MP, et al. Abeta oligomers induce neuronal oxidative stress through an N-methyl-D-aspartate receptor-dependent mechanism that is blocked by the Alzheimer drug memantine. Journal of Biological Chemistry 2007; 282(15): 11590-601.

[4] Melov S, Adlard PA, Morten K, Johnson F, et al. Mitochondrial oxidative stress causes hyperphosphorylation of tau. PLoS One 2007; 2(6): e536.

[5] Su B, Wang X, Lee HG, Tabaton M, Perry G, Smith MA, Zhu X. Chronic oxidative stress causes increased tau phosphorylation in M17 neuroblastoma cells. Neuroscience Letters 2010; 468(3): 267-71.

[6] Wolfe DM, Lee JH, Kumar A, Lee S, Orenstein SJ, Nixon RA. Autophagy failure in Alzheimer's disease and the role of defective lysosomal acidification. European Journal Neuroscience 2013; 37(12): 1949-61.

[7] Martínez E, Navarro A, Ordóñez C, et al. Oxidative stress induces apolipoprotein D overexpression in hippocampus during aging and Alzheimer's disease. Journal of Alzheimer's Disease 2013; 36(1): 129-44.

[8] Tayler H, Fraser T, Miners JS, Kehoe PG, Love S. Oxidative balance in Alzheimer's disease: relationship to APOE, Braak tangle stage, and the concentrations of soluble and insoluble amyloid-β. Journal of Alzheimer's Disease 2010; 22(4): 1363-73.

[9] Mattson MP, Magnus T. Ageing and neuronal vulnerability. Nature Reviews Neuroscience 2006; 7(4): 278-94.

[10] Wang X, Wang W, Li L, Perry G, Lee HG, Zhu X. Oxidative stress and mitochondrial dysfunction in Alzheimer's disease. Biochimica et Biophysica Acta 2014; 1842(8): 1240-7.

[11] Yao J, Irwin RW, Zhao L, Nilsen J, Hamilton RT, Brinton RD. Mitochondrial bioenergetic deficit precedes Alzheimer's pathology in female mouse model of Alzheimer's disease. Proceedings of the National Academy of Science of the United States of America 2009; 106(34): 14670-675.

[12] Yao J, Du H, Yan S, Fang F, et al. Inhibition of amyloid-beta (Abeta) peptide- binding alcohol dehydrogenase-Abeta interaction reduces Abeta accumulation and improves mitochondrial function in a mouse model of Alzheimer's disease. Journal of Neuroscience 2011; 31(6): 2313-20.

[13] Pensalfini A, Zampagni M, Liguri G, Becatti M, et al. Membrane cholesterol enrichment prevents Aβ-induced oxidative stress in Alzheimer's fibroblasts. Neurobiology of Aging 2011; 32(2): 210-22.

[14] Chen Z, Zhong C. Oxidative stress in Alzheimer's disease. Neuroscience Bulletin 2014; 30(2): 271-81.

[15] Schuessel K, Schafer S, Bayer TA, Czech C, et al. Impaired Cu/Zn-SOD activity contributes to increased oxidative damage in APP transgenic mice. Neurobiology of Disease 2005; 18(1): 89-99.

[16] Poppek D, Keck S, Ermak G, et al. Phosphorylation inhibits turnover of the tau protein by the proteasome: influence of RCAN1 and oxidative stress. Biochemical Journal 2006; 400(3): 511-20.

[17] Avila J, Lucas JJ, Perez M, Hernandez F. Role of tau protein in both physiological and pathological conditions. Physiological Reviews 2004; 84(2): 361-84.

[18] Gordon D, Kidd GJ, Smith R. Antisense suppression of tau in cultured rat oligodendrocytes inhibits process formation. Journal of Neuroscience Reseach 2008; 86(12): 2591-601.

[19] Kolarova M, García-Sierra F, Bartos A, Ricny J, Ripova D. Structure and pathology of tau protein in Alzheimer disease. International Journal of Alzheimer's Disease 2012; 2012: 731526.

[20] Fauquant C, Redeker V, Landrieu I, Wieruszeski JM, et al. Systematic identification of tubulin-interacting fragments of the microtubule-associated protein Tau leads to a highly efficient promoter of microtubule assembly. J Biological Chemistry 2011; 286(38): 33358-68.

[21] Li HL, Wang HH, Liu SJ, Deng YQ, Zhang YJ, Tian Q, et al. Phosphorylation of tau antagonizes apoptosis by stabilizing beta-catenin, a mechanism involved in Alzheimer's neurodegeneration. Proceedings of the National Academy of Sciences of the United States of America 2007; 104(9): 3591-96.

[22] Ballatore C, Brunden KR, Huryn DM, Trojanowski JQ, Lee VM, Smith AB 3rd. Microtubule stabilizing agents as potential treatment for Alzheimer's disease and related neurodegenerative tauopathies. Journal of Medicinal Chemistry 2012; 55(21): 8979-96.

[23] Rodríguez-Martín T, Cuchillo-Ibáñez I, Noble W, et al. Tau phosphorylation affects its axonal transport and degradation. Neurobiology of Aging 2013; 34(9): 2146-57.

[24] Simón D, García-García E, Royo F, Falcón-Pérez JM, Avila J. Proteostasis of tau. Tau overexpression results in its secretion via membrane Vesicles. FEBS Letters 2012; 586(1): 47-54.

[25] Iseki E, Yamamoto R, Murayama N, Minegishi M, et al. Immunohisto-chemical investigation of neurofibrillary tangles and their tau isoforms in brains of limbic neurofibrillary tangle dementia. Neuroscience Letters 2006; 405(1-2): 29-33.

[26] Santacruz K, Lewis J, Spires T, et al. Tau suppression in a neurodegenerative mouse model improves memory function. Science 2005; 309(5733): 476-81.

[27] Yoshiyama Y, Lee VM, Trojanowski JQ. Therapeutic strategies for tau mediated neurodegeneration. Journal of Neurology, Neurosurgery and Psychiatry 2013; 84(7): 784-95.

[28] Iijima-Ando K, Zhao L, Gatt A, Shenton C, Iijima K. A DNA damage-activated checkpoint kinase phosphorylates tau and enhances tau-induced neurodegeneration. Human Molecular Genetics 2010; 19(10): 1930-8.

[29] Mendoza J, Sekiya M, Taniguchi T, Iijima KM, Wang R, Ando K. Global Analysis of Phosphorylation of Tau by the Checkpoint Kinases Chk1 and Chk2 in vitro. Journal of Proteome Research 2013; 12(6): 2654-65.

[30] Flunkert S, Hierzer M, Löffler T, Rabl R, Neddens J, et al. Elevated levels of soluble total and hyperphosphorylated tau result in early behavioral deficits and distinct changes in brain pathology in a new tau transgenic mouse model. Neuro-degenerative Diseases 2013; 11(4): 194-205.

[31] Hernandez F, Lucas JJ, Avila J. GSK3 and tau: two convergence points in Alzheimer's disease. Journal of Alzheimer's Disease 2013; 33(Suppl 1): S141-4.

[32] Gao C, Hölscher C, Liu Y, Li L. GSK3: a key target for the development of novel treatments for type 2 diabetes mellitus and Alzheimer disease. Reviews in the Neurosciences 2011; 23(1): 1-11.

[33] Gandy JC, Melendez-Ferro M, Bijur GN, Van Leuven F, et al. Glycogen synthase kinase-3β (GSK3β) expression in a mouse model of Alzheimer's disease: a light and electron microscopy study. Synapse 2013; 67(6): 313-27.

[34] Maldonado H, Ramírez E, Utreras E, Pando ME, Kettlun AM, et al. Inhibition of cyclin-dependent kinase 5 but not of glycogen synthase kinase 3-β prevents neurite retraction andtau hyperphosphorylation caused by secretable products of human T-cell leukemia virus type I-infected lymphocytes. Journal of Neuroscience Research 2011; 89(9): 1489-98.

[35] López-Tobón A, Castro-Álvarez JF, Piedrahita D, Boudreau RL, et al. Silencing of CDK5 as potential therapy for Alzheimer's disease. Reviews in the Neurosciences 2011; 22(2): 143-52.

[36] Corrêa SA, Eales KL. The Role of p38 MAPK and Its Substrates in Neuronal Plasticity and Neurodegenerative Disease. Journal of Signal Transduction 2012; 2012: 649079.

[37] Li G, Yin H, Kuret J. Casein kinase 1 delta phosphorylates tau and disrupts its binding to microtubules. Journal of Biological Chemistry 2004; 279(16): 15938-45.

[38] Liu F, Liang Z, Shi J, Yin D, El-Akkad E, et al. PKA modulates GSK-3β- and cdk5-catalyzed phosphorylation of tau in site- and kinase-specific manners. FEBS Letters 2006; 580(26): 6269-74.

[39] Tsukane M, Yamauchi T. Ca^{2+}/calmodulin-dependent protein kinase II mediates apoptosis of P19 cells expressing human tau during neural differentiation with retinoic acid treatment. Journal of Enzyme Inhibition and Medicinal Chemistry 2009; 24(2): 365-71.

[40] Liu F, Grundke-Iqbal I, Iqbal K, Gong CX. Contributions of protein phosphatases PP1, PP2A, PP2B and PP5 to the regulation of tau phosphorylation. European Journal of Neuroscience 2005; 22(8): 1942-50.

[41] Sanchez-Ortiz E, Hahm BK, Armstrong DL, Rossie S. Protein phosphatase 5 protects neurons against amyloid-beta toxicity. Journal of Neurochemistry 2009; 111 (2): 391-402.

[42] Lubert EJ, Hong Y, Sarge KD. Interaction between protein phosphatase 5 and the A subunit of protein phosphatase 2A: evidence for a heterotrimeric form of protein phosphatase 5. Journal of Biological Chemistry 2001; 276(42): 38582-587.

[43] Landrieu I, Smet-Nocca C, Amniai L, Louis JV, et al. Molecular implication of PP2A and Pin1 in the Alzheimer's disease specific hyperphosphorylation of Tau. PLoS One 2011; 6(6): e21521.

[44] Rudrabhatla P, Pant HC. Role of protein phosphatase 2A in Alzheimer's disease. Current Alzheimer Research 2011; 8(6): 623-32.

[45] Park SS, Jung HJ, Kim YJ, Park TK, et al. Asp664 cleavage of amyloid precursor protein induces tau phosphorylation by decreasing protein phosphatase 2A activity. Journal of Neurochemistry 2012; 123(5): 856-65.

[46] Martin L, Latypova X, Wilson CM, Magnaudeix A, Perrin ML, Terro F. Tau protein phosphatases in Alzheimer's disease: the leading role of PP2A. Ageing Research Reviews 2013; 12(1): 39-49.

[47] Arif M, Wei J, Zhang Q, Liu F, Basurto-Islas G, Grundke-Iqbal I, Iqbal K. Cytoplasmic Retention of Protein Phosphatase 2A-Inhibitor 2 (I2PP2A) Induces Alzheimer-like Abnormal Hyperphosphorylation of Tau. Journal of Biological Chemistry 2014; 289(40): 27677-91.

[48] Arnaud L, Chen S, Liu F, Li B, Khatoon S, Grundke-Iqbal I, Iqbal K.. Mechanism of inhibition of PP2A activity and abnormal hyperphosphorylation of tau by I2(PP2A)/ SET. FEBS Letters 2011; 585(17): 2653-59.

[49] Liu GP, Zhang Y, Yao XQ, Zhang CE, Fang J, Wang Q, Wang JZ. Activation of glycogen synthase kinase-3 inhibits protein phosphatase-2A and the underlying mechanisms. Neurobiology of Aging 2008; 29(9): 1348-58.

[50] Patil S, Chan C. Palmitic and stearic fatty acids induce Alzheimer-like hyperphosphorylation of tau in primary rat cortical neurons. Neuroscience Letters 2005; 384(3): 288-93.

[51] Lovell MA, Xiong S, Xie C, Davies P, Markesbery WR. Induction of hyperphosphorylated tau in primary rat cortical neuron cultures mediated by oxidative stress and glycogen synthase kinase-3. Journal of Alzheimer's Disease 2004 6(6): 659-671.

[52] Zambrano CA, Egaña JT, Núñez MT, et al. Oxidative stress promotes τ dephosphorylation in neuronal cells: the roles of cdk5 and PP1. Free Radical Biology and Medicine 2004; 36(11): 1393-402.

[53] Dias-Santagata D, Fulga TA, Duttaroy A, Feany MB. Oxidative stress mediates tau-induced neurodegeneration in Drosophila. Journal of Clinical Investigation 2007; 117(1): 236-45.

[54] Abou-Sleiman PM, Muqit MM, Wood NW. Expanding insights of mitochondrial dysfunction in Parkinson's disease. Nature Reviews Neuroscience 2006; 7(3): 207-19.

[55] King TD, Clodfelder-Miller B, Barksdale KA, Bijur GN. Unregulated mitochondrial GSK3beta activity results in NADH: ubiquinone oxidoreductase deficiency. Neurotoxicity Research 2008; 14(2): 367-82.

[56] Feng Y, Xia Y, Yu G, Shu X, Ge H, Zeng K, Wang J, Wang X. Cleavage of GSK-3β by calpain counteracts the inhibitory effect of Ser9 phosphorylation on GSK-3β activity induced by H_2O_2. Journal of Neurochemistry 2013; 126(2): 234-42.

[57] Chiara F, Gambalunga A, Sciacovelli M, et al. Chemotherapeutic induction of mitochondrial oxidative stress activates GSK-3α/β and Bax, leading to permeability transition pore opening and tumor cell death. Cell Death and Disease 2012; 3: e444.

[58] Cho MH, Kim DH, Choi JE, et al. Increased phosphorylation of dynamin-related protein 1 and mitochondrial fission in okadaic acid-treated neurons. Brain Research 2012; 1454: 100-110.

[59] Chen L, Liu L, Huang S. Cadmium activates the mitogen-activated protein kinase (MAPK) pathway via induction of reactive oxygen species and inhibition of protein phosphatases 2A and 5. Free Radical Biology and Medicine 2008; 45(7): 1035-44.

[60] Zhang CE, Yang X, Li L, Sui X, et al. Hypoxia-Induced Tau Phosphorylation and Memory Deficit in Rats. Neuro-degenerative Diseases 2014; 14(3): 107-16.

[61] Wade AG, Farmer M, Harari G, et al. Add-on prolonged-release melatonin for cognitive function and sleep in mild to moderate Alzheimer's disease: a 6-month, randomized, placebo-controlled, multicenter trial. Clinical Interventions in Aging 2004; 9: 947-61.

[62] Peng CX, Hu J, Liu D, Hong XP, Wu YY, Zhu LQ, Wang JZ. Disease- modified glycogen synthase kinase-3β intervention by melatonin arrests the pathology and memory deficits in an Alzheimer's animal model. Neurobiology of Aging 2013; 34(6): 1555-63.

[63] Benítez-King G, Ortíz-López L, Jiménez-Rubio G, Ramírez-Rodríguez G. Haloperidol causes cytoskeletal collapse in N1E-115 cells through tau hyperphosphorylation induced by oxidative stress: Implications for neurodevelopment. European Journal of Pharmacology 2010; 644(1-3): 24-31.

[64] Li XC, Wang ZF, Zhang JX, Wang Q, Wang JZ. Effect of melatonin on calyculin A-induced tau hyperphosphorylation. European Journal of Pharmacology 2005; 510(1-2): 25-30.

[65] Hoppe JB, Frozza RL, Horn AP, et al. Amyloid-beta neurotoxicity in organotypic culture is attenuated by melatonin: involvement of GSK-3beta, tau and neuroinflammation. Journal of Pineal Research 2010; 48(3): 230-38.

[66] Lin L, Huang QX, Yang SS, Chu J, Wang JZ, Tian Q. Melatonin in Alzheimer's disease. International Journal of Molecular Sciences 2013; 14(7): 14575-93.

[67] Villaflores OB, Chen YJ, Chen CP, Yeh JM, Wu TY. Effects of curcumin and demethoxy curcumin on amyloid-β precursor and tau proteins through the internal ribosome entry sites: a potential therapeutic for Alzheimer's disease. Taiwan Journal of Obstetrics and Gynecology 2012; 51(4): 554-64.

[68] Ma QL, Zuo X, Yang F, Ubeda OJ, et al. Curcumin suppresses soluble tau dimers and corrects molecular chaperone, synaptic, and behavioral deficits in aged human tau transgenic mice. Journal of Biological Chemistry 2013; 288(6): 4056-65.

[69] Patil SP, Tran N, Geekiyanage H, Liu L, Chan C. Curcumin-induced upregulation of the anti-tau cochaperone BAG2 in primary rat cortical neurons. Neuroscience Letters 2013; 554: 121-5.

[70] Stuerenburg HJ, Ganzer S, Müller-Thomsen T. Plasma beta carotene in Alzheimer's disease. Association with cerebrospinal fluid beta-amyloid 1-40, (Abeta40), beta-amyloid 1-42 (Abeta42) and total Tau. Neuro Endocrinology Letters 2005; 26(6): 696-8.

[71] Chen Y, Wang C, Hu M, et al. Effects of ginkgolide A on okadaic acid- induced tau hyperphosphorylation and the PI3K-Akt signaling pathway in N2a cells. Planta Medica 2012; 78(12): 1337-41.

[72] Galasko DR, Peskind E, Clark CM, et al. Antioxidants for Alzheimer disease: a randomized clinical trial with cerebrospinal fluid biomarker measures. Archives of Neurology 2012; 69(7): 836-41.

[73] Cente M, Filipcik P, Mandakova S, Zilka N, Krajciova G, Novak M. Expression of a truncated human tau protein induces aqueous-phase free radicals in a rat model of tauopathy: implications for targeted antioxidative therapy. Journal of Alzheimer's Disease 2009; 17(4): 913-920.

[74] Yoon I, Lee KH, Cho J. Gossypin protects primary cultured rat cortical cells from oxidative stress and beta-amyloid-induced toxicity. Archives of Pharmacal Research 2004; 27(4): 454-59.

[75] Funderburk SF, Marcellino BK, Yue Z. Cell "self-eating" (autophagy) mechanism in Alzheimer's disease. Mount Sinai Journal of Medicine 2010; 77(1): 59- 68.

[76] Bové J, Martínez-Vicente M, Vila M. Fighting neurodegeneration with rapamycin: mechanistic insights. Nature Reviews Neuroscience 2011; 12(8): 437-52.

[77] Cai Z, Yan LJ. Rapamycin, Autophagy and Alzheimer's Disease. Journal of Biochemical and Pharmacological Research 2013; 1(2): 84-90.

[78] Dunlop EA, Tee AR. The kinase triad, AMPK, mTORC1 and ULK1, maintains energy and nutrient homoeostasis. Biochemical Society Transactions 2013; 41(4): 939-43.

[79] Ishizuka Y, Kakiya N, Witters LA et al. AMP-activated protein kinase counteracts brain-derived neurotrophic factor-induced mammalian target of rapamycin complex 1 signaling in neurons. Journal of Neurochemistry 2013; 127(1): 66-77.

[80] Jung CH, Seo M, Otto NM, Kim DH. ULK1 inhibits the kinase activity of mTORC1 and cell proliferation. Autophagy 2011; 7(10): 1212-21.

[81] Maiuri MC, Malik SA, Morselli E, Kepp O, et al. Stimulation of autophagy by the p53 target gene Sestrin2. Cell Cycle 2009; 8(10): 1571-6.

[82] Chan EY, Longatti A, McKnight NC, Tooze SA. Kinase-inactivated ULK proteins inhibit autophagy via their conserved C-terminal domains using an Atg13-independent mechanism. Molecular and Cellular Biology 2009; 29(1): 157-71.

[83] Sarkar S, Floto RA, Berger Z, Imarisio S, Cordenier A, Pasco M, Cook LJ, Rubinsztein DC. Lithium induces autophagy by inhibiting inositol monophosphatase. Journal of Cell Biology 2005; 170(7): 1101-11.

[84] Zou J, Yue F, Jiang X, Li W, Yi J, Liu L. Mitochondrion-associated protein LRPPRC suppresses the initiation of basal levels of autophagy via enhancing Bcl-2 stability. Biochemical Journal 2013; 454(3): 447-57.

[85] Alirezaei M, Kiosses WB, Fox HS. Decreased neuronal autophagy in HIV dementia: a mechanism of indirect neurotoxicity. Autophagy 2008; 4(7): 963-6.

[86] Shpilka T, Weidberg H, Pietrokovski S, Elazar Z. Atg8: an autophagy-related ubiquitin-like protein family. Genome Biology 2011; 12(7): 226.

[87] Kang R, Zeh HJ, Lotze MT, Tang D. The Beclin 1 network regulates autophagy and apoptosis. Cell Death and Differentiation 2011; 18(4): 571-80.

[88] Lünemann JD, Schmidt J, Schmid D, Barthel K, et al. Beta-amyloid is a substrate of autophagy in sporadic inclusion body myositis. Annals of Neurology 2007; 61(5): 476-483.

[89] Jaeger PA, Pickford F, Sun CH, Lucin KM, Masliah E, Wyss-Coray T. Regulation of amyloid precursor protein processing by the Beclin 1 complex. PLoS One 2010; 5(6): e11102.

[90] Ma JF, Huang Y, Chen SD, Halliday G. Immunohistochemical evidence for macroautophagy in neurones and endothelial cells in Alzheimer's disease. Neuropathology and Applied Neurobiology 2010; 36(4): 312-19.

[91] Yu WH, Cuervo AM, Kumar A, Peterhoff CM, Schmidt SD, et al. Macroautophagy - a novel Beta-amyloid peptide-generating pathway activated in Alzheimer's disease. Journal of Cell Biology 2005; 171(1): 87-98.

[92] Perucho J, Casarejos MJ, Gomez A, Solano RM, et al. Trehalose protects from aggravation of amyloid pathology induced by isoflurane anesthesia in APP(swe) mutant mice. Current Alzheimer Research 2012; 9(3): 334-43.

[93] Lai AY, McLaurin J. Inhibition of amyloid-beta peptide aggregation rescues the autophagic deficits in the TgCRND8 mouse model of Alzheimer disease. Biochimica et Biophysica Acta 2012; 1822(10): 1629-37.

[94] Nixon RA, Yang DS, Lee JH. Neurodegenerative lysosomal disorders: a continuum from development to late age. Autophagy 2008; 4(5): 590-9.

[95] Wei J, Fujita M, Nakai M, Waragai M, Sekigawa A, et al. Protective role of endogenous gangliosides for lysosomal pathology in a cellular model of synucleinopathies. American Journal of Pathology 2009; 174(5): 1891-909.

[96] Cardoso SM, Pereira CF, Moreira PI, Arduino DM, Esteves AR, Oliveira CR. Mitochondrial control of autophagic lysosomal pathway in Alzheimer's disease. Experimental Neurology 2010; 223(2): 294-8.

[97] Silva DF, Esteves AR, Arduino DM, Oliveira CR, Cardoso SM. Amyloid-β- induced mitochondrial dysfunction impairs the autophagic lysosomal pathway in a tubulin dependent pathway. Journal of Alzheimer's Disease 2011; 26(3): 565-81.

[98] Wang Y, Mandelkow E. Degradation of tau protein by autophagy and proteasomal pathways. Biochemical Society Transactions 2012; 40(4): 644-52.

[99] Caccamo A, Magrì A, Medina DX, Wisely EV, et al. mTOR regulates tau phosphorylation and degradation: implications for Alzheimer's disease and other tauopathies. Aging Cell 2013; 12(3): 370-80.

[100] Liu Y, Su Y, Wang J, Sun S, Wang T, Qiao X, Run X, Li H, Liang Z. Rapamycin decreases tau phosphorylation at Ser214 through regulation of cAMP-dependent kinase. Neurochemistry International 2013; 62(4): 458-67.

[101] Ozcelik S, Fraser G, Castets P, Schaeffer V, Skachokova Z, et al. Rapamycin attenuates the progression of tau pathology in P301S tau transgenic mice. PLoS One 2013; 8(5): e62459.

[102] Dolan PJ, Johnson GV. A caspase cleaved form of tau is preferentially degraded through the autophagy pathway. Journal of Biological Chemistry 2010; 285(29): 21978-87.

[103] Krüger U, Wang Y, Kumar S, Mandelkow EM. Autophagic degradation of tau in primary neurons and its enhancement by trehalose. Neurobiology of Aging 2012; 33(10): 2291-305.

[104] Kim SI, Lee WK, Kang SS, Lee SY, et al. Suppression of autophagy and activation of glycogen synthase kinase 3beta facilitate the aggregate formation of tau. Korean Journal of Physiology and Pharmacology 2011; 15(2): 107-14.

[105] Lim F, Hernández F, Lucas JJ, Gómez-Ramos P, Morán MA, Avila J. FTDP-17 mutations in tau transgenic mice provoke lysosomal abnormalities and Tau filaments in forebrain. Molecular and Cellular Neurosciences 2001; 18(6): 702-14.

[106] Lin WL, Lewis J, Yen SH, Hutton M, Dickson DW. Ultrastructural neuronal pathology in transgenic mice expressing mutant (P301L) human tau. Journal of Neurocytology 2003; 32(9): 1091-105.

[107] Magnaudeix A, Wilson CM, Page G, Bauvy C, Codogno P, et al. PP2A blockade inhibits autophagy and causes intraneuronal accumulation of ubiquitinated proteins. Neurobiology of Aging 2013; 34(3): 770-90.

[108] Yoon SY, Choi JE, Kweon HS, Choe H, et al. Okadaic acid increases autophagosomes in rat neurons: implications for Alzheimer's disease. Journal of Neuroscience Research 2008; 86(14): 3230-9.

[109] Hamano T, Gendron TF, Causevic E, Yen SN, et al. Autophagic-lysosomal perturbation enhances tau aggregation in transfectants with induced wild-type tau expression. European Journal of Neuroscience 2008; 27(5): 1119-30.

[110] Wang Y, Martinez-Vicente M, Kruger U, Kaushik S, Wong E, Mandelkow EM, Cuervo AM, Mandelkow E. (2009). Tau fragmentation, aggregation and clearance: the dual role of lysosomal processing. Human Molecular Genetics 2009; 18(21): 4153-70.

[111] Inoue K, Rispoli J, Kaphzan H, Klann E, et al. Macroautophagy deficiency mediates age-dependent neurodegeneration through a phospho-tau pathway. Molecular Neurodegeneration 2012; 7: 48.

6

The Mevalonate Pathway in Alzheimer's Disease — Cholesterol and Non-Sterol Isoprenoids

Amany Mohamed, Kevan Smith and Elena Posse de Chaves

Additional information is available at the end of the chapter

1. Introduction

The brain is a lipid-rich organ, with approximately 50% of its dry mass constituted by lipids [1]. The main lipid in the brain is cholesterol. The human brain represents only 2% of the total body mass but contains 25% of the total body cholesterol [2, 3]. Therefore, it is not surprising that lipids have important functions in the brain and that dysregulation of brain lipid metabolism has been linked to brain diseases, in particular Alzheimer's disease (AD). The interest in understanding the link between lipids and AD pathology has increased dramatically since the 1990s, when it was discovered that the isoform 4 (ε4) of the cholesterol transport protein apolipoprotein E, is a major risk factor for AD development [4]. Since then an important body of evidence derived from genetic, epidemiological, and biochemical studies has identified the role of cholesterol in many critical aspects of AD neuropathology. The finding that a number of genes involved in cholesterol homeostasis represent susceptibility loci for sporadic or late-onset AD (reviewed in [5-9]), and the evidence that alterations in cholesterol homeostasis are significant in regulation of Aβ production, formation of amyloid plaques, tau hyperphosphorylation, Aβ toxicity, and other mechanisms (reviewed in [5, 10-12]) highlight the importance of the dysregulation of cholesterol homeostasis in AD. [7, 9, 13-20]. Cholesterol homeostasis disturbances in AD may be both consequences of the neurodegenerative process and contributors to the pathogenesis.

2. Cholesterol homeostasis in the brain

Cholesterol homeostasis is the balance between synthesis and uptake, and efflux and metabolism. In the brain, this process acquires peculiar characteristics because of differences in the ability of neurons and glia to perform each of these processes (Figure 1).

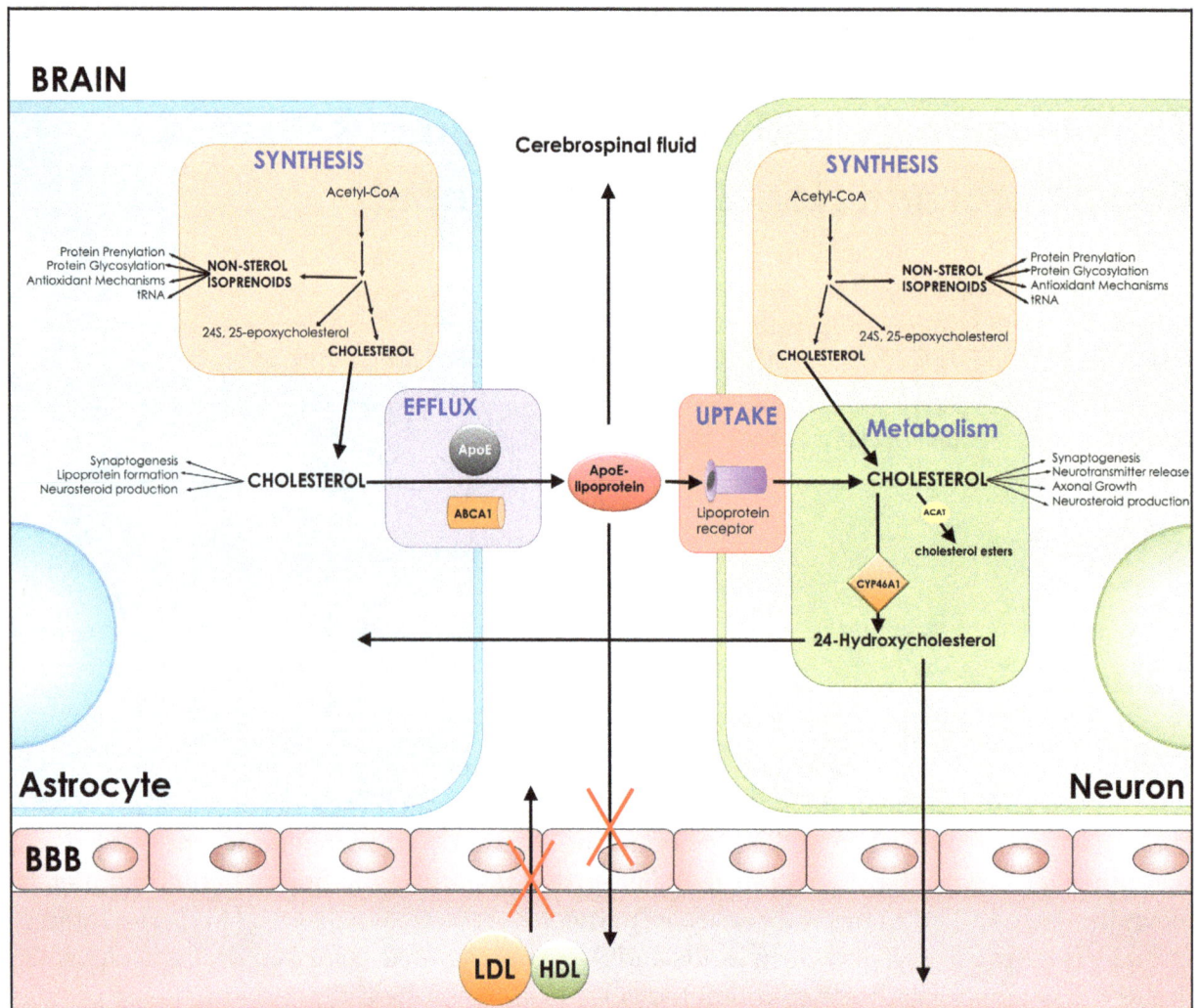

Figure 1. Cholesterol homeostasis in the brain. Cellular cholesterol is synthesized from acetyl-CoA in a multistep mevalonate pathway. Cholesterol and Apo-E synthesized in astrocytes are secreted in an ABCA1-dependent process, forming discoidal lipoprotein particles, which can be further lipidated. Brain lipoproteins are delivered to the CSF. Apo-E is a ligand for LDLR family members, which mediate neuronal lipoprotein uptake, thereby providing a supply of cholesterol to neurons. Excess cholesterol is metabolized to 24-hydroxycholesterol, which crosses the BBB and passes into the circulation. A small part of cholesterol (~1%) is esterified by ACAT. Only insignificant amounts of plasma HDL or LDL cross the BBB under normal conditions.

Cholesterol synthesis is crucial in the brain because the brain is separated from the peripheral pool of cholesterol by the blood brain barrier (BBB), which, under normal conditions, is impermeable to plasma lipoproteins [2, 3]. Thus, brain cholesterol originates almost exclusively from *de novo* biosynthesis through the mevalonate pathway. Cholesterol synthesis *in situ* in the brain is very active in order to meet the brain demands. Cholesterol is essential for normal synaptogenesis and plays important roles in axonal development, neurotransmitter release and neurosteroid production [2, 21]. Brain cholesterol synthesis is sufficient to meet the demands during development and in adult life, although this local synthesis decreases with age [22]. Genetic defects in enzymes involved in cholesterol synthesis cause severe neurological abnormalities underscoring the importance of endogenous cholesterol synthesis for normal brain function [23, 24]. The identity of the cells responsible for cholesterol synthesis in the adult brain is still a matter of debate. Neurons have a lower rate of cholesterol synthesis than astrocytes [25] and outsource cholesterol from astrocytes to form and maintain axons, dendrites and synapses [21, 26, 27]. In fact, based on the discovery that suppression of cholesterol synthesis in vivo in adult cerebellar neurons did not affect the viability of the neurons or the shape and density of synapses [28], it was suggested that neurons do not require autonomous cholesterol synthesis and are minor contributors to adult brain cholesterol synthesis [28]. However, *in situ* hybridization demonstrated that transcripts of several enzymes involved in cholesterol synthesis localize specifically to neurons in pyramidal and granular layers of mouse hippocampus [29], indicating that some adult neurons maintain the ability to synthesize cholesterol. Yet, there is ample evidence that brain neurons utilize cholesterol derived from astrocytes. Astrocytes provide cholesterol to neurons via apolipo-protein-mediated efflux and formation of HDL-like particles containing apoE [27]. Adenosine triphosphate-binding cassette (ABC) transporters, mainly ABCA1, mediate lipidation of nascent lipoproteins [30]. Neurons import cholesterol via lipoprotein receptor-mediated endocytosis [31]. Astrocyte-secreted lipoproteins are delivered to the CSF but they don't cross the BBB [32, 33].

Neurons convert excess cholesterol into a more polar metabolite that crosses the BBB, 24 (S) hydroxycholesterol (24-HC) by the enzyme cholesterol 24-hydroxylase (CYP46A1) [34, 35]. CYP46A1 is selectively expressed in the brain [36], in particular in pyramidal neurons of the hippocampus and cortex and in Purkinje cells in cerebellum, but not in astrocytes [25, 37]. 24-HC is a very important regulator of the mevalonate pathway (Section 3). In addition, 24-HC regulates cholesterol efflux in astrocytes [38]. Cholesterol also undergoes esterification catalyzed by the enzyme acyl CoA-cholesterol acyltransferase (ACAT) [39]. Although cholesterol esterification is not a major metabolic process in the brain, and cholesterol esters represent only 1% of the total cholesterol content in brains of human [40] and mice [41], ACAT has been identified as a crucial enzyme in AD [42].

Cholesterol-related genes that have been associated with AD encode primarily, components of the glia/neuron cholesterol shuttle processes, including apoE [4, 43], the apolipoprotein clusterin [44], ABCA1 [45-48], CYP46A1 [49-52], several members of the LDL receptor family [53-55], and ACAT [56]. Much less information is available with respect to the genetic association of AD with genes of enzymes of the mevalonate pathway. The few studies available did not provide strong associations. Thus, it is likely that changes in the mevalonate pathway identified in AD are a consequence of the disease. Here we focus on the evidence that indicate that the mevalonate pathway "per se" is affected in AD.

3. The mevalonate pathway in the brain and in AD

The brain produces cholesterol and a number of non-sterol isoprenoids such as farnesylpyrophosphate (FPP), geranylgeranylpyrophosphate (GGPP), ubiquinone and dolichol, exclusively through the mevalonate pathway. The mevalonate pathway comprises successive enzymatic reactions that convert acetyl-CoA into the different final sterol and non-sterol products [57, 58]. For the purposes of the discussion we have separated the mevalonate pathway in components: pre-squalene pathway, post-squalene pathway, shunt pathway and non-sterols isoprenoids pathway (Figure 2). The kinetics of the enzymes involved in the mevalonate pathway have been thoroughly studied [58, 59]. Enzymes of the mevalonate pathway are expressed in the brain of rodents and humans [29, 60] and the expression of many of them is developmentally regulated in the brain [61, 62]. Inborn defects in enzymes of the mevalonate pathway result in structural abnormalities of the brain and may be accompanied by neurodevelopmental/behavioral defects [63].

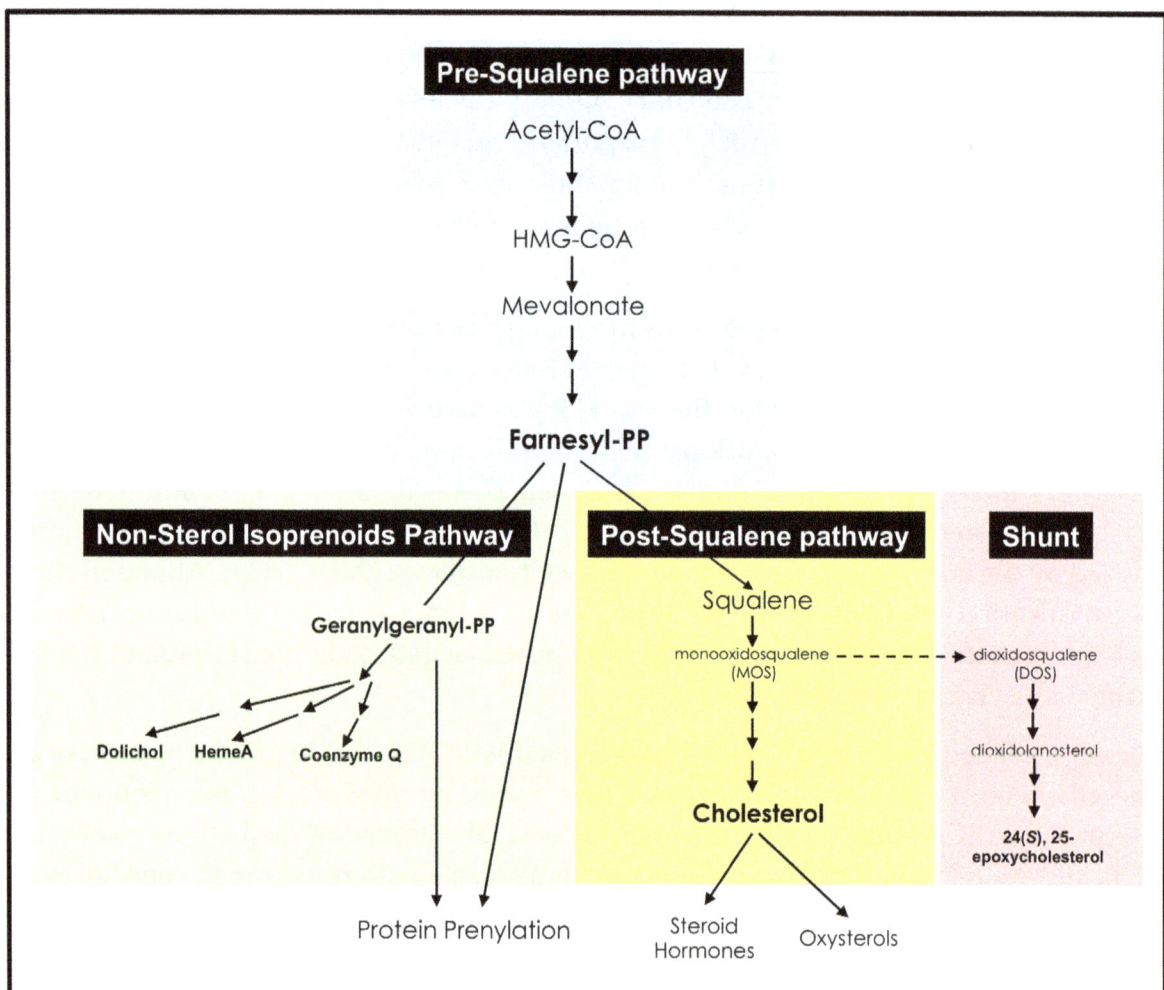

Figure 2. The mevalonate pathway. The mevalonate pathway has been divided in different components to facilitate the understanding of its regulation.

There is only limited information of changes in the mevalonate pathway enzymes and lipid intermediates in AD brains, although certain exceptions exist. The lipid products of the mevalonate pathway seem to be regulated highly individually in AD, likely through post-translational modifications of the enzymes and/or changes in levels of substrates. Most of the studies on the mevalonate pathway in AD have focused on cholesterol, although more recent work has also paid attention to the non-sterol isoprenoid branch of the pathway. In this chapter we focused on studies performed in brains and brain cells although there is important evidence that changes in plasma cholesterol levels may be relevant to AD development and/or progression [64]. The interest in understanding the role of the mevalonate pathway in AD increased with the reports that patients taking statins had lower incidence of AD than the general population [13-17, 65]. More recent prospective studies have produced conflicting results on the matter [15-19]. This is still an area of intense research and debate.

The mevalonate pathway is tightly regulated at the transcriptional and post-transcriptional levels to avoid accumulation of cholesterol while maintaining proper supply of non-sterol isoprenoids.

3.1. Regulation of the mevalonate pathway by SREBP-2 and LXR

Transcriptional regulation of the mevalonate pathway is mediated by two main transcription factors namely sterol-regulatory element binding protein type-2 (SREBP-2) and liver X receptors (LXR). SREBP-2 belongs to a family of membrane-bound transcription factors that regulate cholesterol and fatty acid homeostasis. Studies in knockout and transgenic mice demonstrated that cholesterol synthesis is preferentially regulated by SREBP-2 [66, 67]. SREBP-2 is synthesized and inserted in the endoplasmic reticulum (ER) as an inactive precursor (P)SREBP-2 [68]. (P)SREBP-2 has two transmembrane helices with the N- and C- terminals projecting into the cytosol [68]. The C-terminus of (P)SREBP-2 interacts with C-terminus of SREBP cleavage-activating protein (SCAP), a sterol-regulated escort protein. SCAP has eight transmembrane helices, of which transmembrane helices 2-6 are defined as a sterol sensing domain [68, 69]. (P)SREBP-2-SCAP complex has to be transported into coat protein complex II (COPII) vesicles that bud from the ER and travel to the Golgi complex [70]. Mice with haploinsufficiency of SCAP in the brain had reduced SREBP-2 processing and reduced SREBP-2 expression. Consequently, reduced SCAP level resulted in decreased expression of many enzymes in the mevalonate pathway and 30% reduction in cholesterol synthesis leading to impaired synaptic transmission and cognitive deficits [71]. At the Golgi, sequential proteolytic cleavage of (P)SREBP-2 by Site-1-protease (S1P) [72] and Site-2-protease (S2P) [73] releases the N-terminal/mature/nuclear SREBP-2 ((M)SREBP-2) that enters the nucleus to regulate gene transcription [66, 68, 74]. In the nucleus, (M)SREBP-2 binds to sterol regulatory elements (SREs) in the promoter of target genes in order to regulate gene expression [68]. SREBPs alone are relatively weak activators of gene expression. Transcriptional activities of SREBPs are highly enhanced by other cofactors such as nuclear factor Y(NF-Y) [75] and specificity protein-1 (sp-1) [76] or by the presence of two SRE motifs as in genes encoding enzymes such as 3-hydroxy-3-methylglutarylCoA reductase (HMGCR), squalene synthase [75] and 24-dihydrocholesterol reductase (DHCR24) [77]. (M)SREBP-2 increases the expression of most enzymes involved in the mevalonate pathway and the expression of LDLR involved in exogenous cholesterol uptake [66, 67]. In addition, SREBP-2 increases the expression of miR33a (encoded by an intron of SREBP-2) and miR128-2. miR33a and miR128-2 block ABCA1 and ABCG1 expression reducing cholesterol efflux [78-84]. High level of (M)SREBP-2 were detected in pyramidal neurons in hippocampus and cerebral neocotex of normal rat brain [85]. The main regulator of SREBP-2 proteolytic processing is cholesterol. When ER cholesterol falls below 5% of total ER lipids (molar basis), SREBP-2 cleavage is activated [86]. On the other hand, when cholesterol accumulates at the ER, it binds to SCAP inducing a conformational change that promotes SCAP binding to ER integral membrane proteins Insulin-Induced gene-1 or 2 (Insig-1 and Insig- 2) [87, 88]. Once bound to Insigs, SCAP is unable to bind to COPII and the SCAP-(P)SREBP-2 complex is not transported to the Golgi leading to reduced SREBP-2 processing [89]. In vitro experiments revealed that cholesterol, and the cholesterol precursors desmosterol and 7-DHC, but not lanosterol or oxysterols are able to change SCAP conformation [87]. Desmosterol and cholesterol bind to SCAP in a similar manner [88, 90, 91]. Oxysterols also reduce SREBP-2 processing but they do so by binding directly to Insigs and not to SCAP [92]. SREBP-2 positively regulates its own expression via binding to SRE in the promoter of its own gene [93]. It also increases expression of specific miRNAs for negative SREBP-2 regulators such as miR-182, which reduce expression of Fbxw7, an E3 ubiquitin ligase involved in nuclear SREBP-2 degradation and miR-96, which targets Insig-2 [94]. Therefore, miR-182 and miR-96 increase SREBP-2 processing, reduce its degradation and consequently enhance its transcriptional activity.

LXRs (LXRα and LXRβ) also play a role in the regulation of the mevalonate pathway by activating or inhibiting expression of enzymes of the mevalonate pathway (reviewed in [95]). LXR are ligand-activated transcription factors belonging to the nuclear hormone receptor superfamily [96, 97]. Expression level of LXRα in the brain is much lower than in the liver, however, LXRβ is highly expressed in the brain compared to the liver [98]. SREBP-2 and LXR work in harmony in order to regulate the mevalonate pathway. SREBP-2 activation will enhance cholesterol production and consequently oxysterol production, leading to LXR activation and LXR targets expression [99]. On the other hand, LXRs activation enhances cholesterol efflux, reduces cellular cholesterol uptake [100, 101] and suppresses the expression of some enzymes in the post-squalene mevalonate pathway [102]. Consequently, LXR activation will reduce cellular cholesterol level leading to SREBP-2 processing and activation. In accordance, synthetic LXR agonist GW683965A significantly increased SREBP-2, LDLR, and HMGCR expression in astrocytes by indirect mechanims [38]. Moreover, significantly reduced number of SREBP-2 and HMGCR transcripts were detected in brains of LXRα and β null mice [103].

3.1.1. Transcriptional regulation of the mevalonate pathway by SREBP-2 in AD

Transcription factor profiling showed no difference in SREBPs between non-demented and AD brain cortical samples [104], however it was not discriminated if the probe was for SREBP-2 or SREBP-1. In autopsied hippocampus of patients with incipient AD, SREBF-1 was found to be elevated [105]. Haploinsufficiency of Scap, a key regulator of SREBP-2, in mice brain resulted in impaired synaptic transmission, as measured by decreased paired pulse facilitation and long-term potentiation; and was associated with behavioral and cognitive changes [71], suggesting that down-regulation of the mevalonate pathway may play an important role in the increased rates of cognitive decline in AD. Studies at the subcellular level suggest that SREBP-2 may be posttranslationally regulated in AD. We demonstrated that oAβ$_{42}$ inhibit

SREBP-2 maturation in cultured neurons [106]. We also discovered that the levels of (M)SREBP-2 are reduced in the frontal cortex of the AD CRND8 mouse [107], suggesting that the negative regulation of SREBP-2 may also occur *in vivo* in AD. Recently, it was reported that APP also controls neuronal cholesterol synthesis through the SREBP pathway [108]. These studies showed that APP levels inversely correlate with SREBP in mice and man, and demonstrated that inhibition of the mevalonate pathway by APP impairs neuronal activity. The interaction of APP and SREBP-1 in the Golgi prevented the release of mature SREBP-1 and the translocation of SREBP-1 to the nucleus. Our data, on the other hand, indicated that $A\beta_{42}$ did not affect the enzymatic cleavage of SREBP-2 "per se" nor did it block mature SREBP-2 translocation to the nucleus, but impaired the delivery of SREBP-2 to the Golgi preventing cleavage of (P)SREBP-2 [107]. Interestingly, the regulation of SREBP by APP takes place preferentially in neurons. In astrocytes, APP and SREBP1 did not interact nor did APP affect cholesterol biosynthesis, but neuronal expression of APP decreased both HMGCR and cholesterol 24-hydroxylase mRNA levels leading to inhibition of neuronal activity [108].

3.2. Pre-squalene pathway

The pre-squalene mevalonate pathway is depicted in Figure 3. Acetoacetyl Co-A is formed from two moles of acetyl Co-A in the presence of acetoacetyl Co-A thiolase. 3-hydroxy-3-methylglutaryl (HMG) Co-A is formed from one mole of acetyl Co-A and acetoacetyl Co-A in the presence of HMG Co-A synthase (HMGS). HMGCR converts HMG Co-A to mevalonic acid [109]. The rate-limiting enzyme of the pathway is HMGCR [110], one of the most highly regulated enzymes in nature [111]. In human brains HMGCR expression was demonstrated in both neurons and glia [112]. Studies in adult mouse brain tissue showed HMGCR expression within cortical, hippocampal, and basal forebrain cholinergic neurons [29, 60]. HMGCR protein and activity are localized in the ER and peroxisomes in the CNS [113] and in other organs. Due to the critical function of this enzyme early in the mevalonate pathway, there are no human syndromes known to be associated with HMGCR loss of function, and mouse embryos homozygous for the Hmgcr knockout allele do not progress beyond the blastocyst stage. On the other hand mice heterozygous for the Hmgcr mutation showed normal development, gross anatomy, and fertility (reviewed in [114]). HMGCR is the target of statins.

The product of HMGCR, mevalonic acid, is phosphorylated sequentially to 5-phosphomevalonate by the enzyme mevalonate kinase (MK) and to 5-pyrophosphomevalonate by phosphomevalonate kinase (PMK). MK is the second essential enzyme of the isoprenoid/cholesterol biosynthetic pathway [115]. Inherited mutations in human MK are correlated with two diseases characterized by neurological dysfunction namely mevalonic aciduria and Hyper-IgD syndrome (reviewed in [114, 116]).

5-Pyrophosphomevalonate is converted to isopentenylpyrophosphate (IPP) by mevalonate diphosphate decarboxylase. IPP is required for synthesis of all further products of the mevalonate pathway [117]. IPP is isomerized to dimethylallyl pyrophosphate (DMPP) in the presence of IPP isomerase (IPPI) [58, 118].

IPP and/or DMPP are required for isopentenylation, which is an essential modification of specialized tRNA that transfers the amino acid selenocysteine (tRNA[Sec]) [119, 120]. Selenopro-

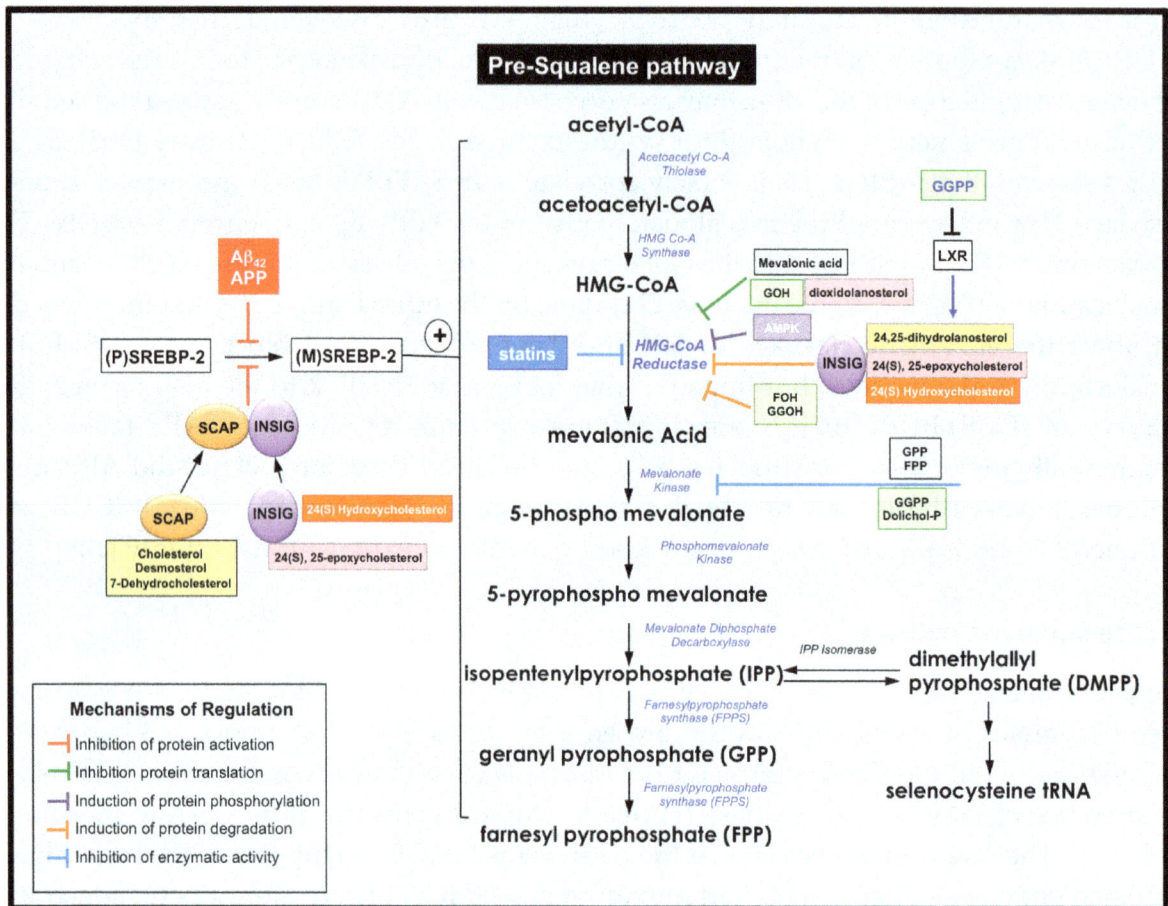

Figure 3. The pre-squalene pathway. Schematic representation of the pre-squalene mevalonate pathway and key enzymes regulating FPP synthesis. The rate-limiting enzyme of the pathway is HMGCR. Several regulatory feedback mechanisms exist at the level of many enzymes of the pathway.

teins have been implicated in protein folding, degradation of misfolded membrane proteins, and control of cellular calcium homeostasis, all processes known to be dysfunctional in neurodegenerative diseases [121, 122]. Moreover, neuron-specific ablation of selenoprotein expression causes a neurodevelopmental and neurodegenerative phenotype affecting the cerebral cortex and hippocampus [123]; and impaired expression of selenoproteins in the brain triggers striatal neuronal loss leading to coordination defects in mice [124]. Statins, by reducing production of IPP, interfere with the enzymatic isopentenylation of tRNA[Sec] and prevent its maturation to a functional tRNA molecule, resulting in the reduction of the expression of selenoproteins [125]. Other functions of IPP include its antinociceptive effect, mediated by inhibition of transient receptor potential (TRP)-channels, TRPV3 and TRPA1 [126]. Interestingly, DMPP has effects on TRP- channels opposites to those of IPP, inducing enhanced acute pain behavior [127].

IPP combines with DMPP to form geranyl pyrophosphate (GPP); and GPP is condensed with another molecule of IPP to yield farnesylpyrophosphate (FPP). GPP and FPP syntheses are catalyzed by farnesylpyrophosphate synthase (FPPS), a prenyltranferase [128-130]. FPP initiates the branches of the pathway that generate cholesterol and non-sterol isoprenoids.

3.2.1. Regulation of enzymes of the pre-squalene pathway

HMGCR is the rate-limiting enzyme of the mevalonate pathway. HMGCR is transcriptionally activated by SREBP-2 [131]. The presence of two SRE motifs in HMGCR promoter leads to a higher level sterol-dependent regulation [75]. Gene regulation by the SREBP pathway is slow and its down-regulation requires several hours to effectively decrease mRNA of target genes [132]. In order to accomplish a rapid (within 1 h) switch off of cholesterol synthesis HMGCR is extensively regulated at the translational and posttranslational levels (Figure 3). HMGCR is post-transcriptionally regulated by alternative splicing/skipping of exon 13 leading to production of a shorter unproductive transcript that encodes an inactive enzyme. In the liver, HMGCR alternative splicing is regulated by sterols (cholesterol and 25-hydroxycholesterol), so sterol accumulation increases the proportion of shorter transcript and vice versa. Interestingly, sterol-mediated alternative splicing of HMGCR occurs faster than sterol-mediated transcriptional inhibition of HMGCR [133]. Mevalonate and certain downstream derivatives such as dioxidolanosterol (a shunt pathway intermediate) and GOH regulate HMGCR mRNA translation reducing its rate of synthesis [134-137]. Mevalonate has been shown to change polysome distribution of HMGCR mRNA leading to inhibition of HMGCR translation at the initiation step [138]. HMGCR is post-translationally regulated via phosphorylation and ubiquitin/proteasomal degradation. Short-term regulation of HMGCR is mediated via phosphorylation by AMPK and dephosphorylation by PP2A (protein phosphatase 2A). HMGCR exists in the cell in both unphosphorylated (active) and phosphorylated (inactive) states [139-141]. As a master regulator of cellular energy homeostasis, AMPK phosphorylates HMGCR to inhibit cholesterol synthesis, an energy intensive process. The implications of AMPK-mediated regulation of HMGCR are controversial. In mutant Drosophila lacking functional AMPK, higher activity of HMGCR and consequent higher rate of the mevalonate pathway were associated with progressive neurodegeneration [142]. On the other hand, activation of AMPK by quercetin reduced HMGCR activity, cholesterol synthesis and enhanced cognitive functions in high cholesterol fed old mice [143]. The best understood mechanism of HMGCR post transcriptional regulation is the sterol-mediated ubiquitination and proteasomal degradation. This mechanism requires binding of HMGCR to Insig-1 or Insig-2 and recruitment of Ring-finger ubiquitin ligases, Gp78, Trc8, and MARCH6 [144-146]. Insig binds to the sterol-sensing domain in HMGCR [147]. HMGCR share many sequence similarities in the sterol-sensing domain with SCAP, thus Insigs can bind with both HMGCR and SCAP [148]. The binding of Insigs has radically different consequences for SCAP and HMGCR. Upon binding Insig, HMGCR is ubiquitinated and degraded [147, 149], whereas, as indicated above SCAP is retained in the ER [89]. Both processes inhibit the mevalonate pathway. The oxysterols 25-EC (synthesized by the shunt pathway, Section 3.3.1.) and 24-HC; and the post-squalene intermediate 24, 25-dihydrolanosterol (Section 3.3.0), but not cholesterol, bind to Insigs and induce HMGCR degradation [91, 150-152]. Indeed, it is the accumulation of 24, 25-dihydrolanosterol the mechanism by which LXRα enhances HMGCR [102]. Adding an additional level of regulation, the non-sterol isoprenoid GGPP antagonizes LXR, blocking HMGCR degradation [153, 154]. Studies in vitro suggested that two metabolites of the non-sterol isoprenoids pathway namely farnesol (FOH) and geranylgeranyol (GGOH) enhance HMGCR degradation beyond the effect elicited by sterols. FOH and GGOH do not target the interaction between Insigs and HMGCR but seem to rely on protein prenylation [147, 155-158]. Consequently, a GGPP synthase (GGPPS) inhibitor, and a geranylgeranyl transferase I (GGTaseI) inhibitor prevented the enhancement of HMGCR degradation [155].

MK is regulated transcriptionally by SREBP-2 through an SRE in its promoter (Horton 2002). MK activity is post-translationally reduced by GGPP, FPP, GPP and dolichol phosphate via competitive inhibition at ATP binding site [159, 160]. GGPP is the strongest inhibitor of MK activity.

3.2.2. Pre-squalene mevalonate pathway in AD

Information on the status and regulation of HMGCR in AD is very limited. HMGCR is the most important enzyme of the pre-squalene mevalonate pathway. No changes in gene expression of HMGCR were found in AD brain in humans and in a mouse model of AD [161]. Genetic association of HMGCR was found in patients under the age of 75 [162], and HMGCR promoter polymorphisms alone or with polymorphisms in other proteins of cholesterol homeostasis were associated with AD risk and cognitive deterioration in some studies [163, 164], but not in all populations [165]. The AlzGene meta-analysis for HMGCR is negative [7]. Poirier's group identified HMGCR as a genetic modifier for risk, age of onset and mild cognitive impairment (MCI) conversion to AD. In their recent study they found that carriers of a specific variant of HMGCR display a protective effect that resembled in size and gender to what has been reported for APOE2 in humans [166]. Information on protein HMGCR levels and activity in the carriers' brains is expected to be available soon. Age- and sex-dependent dysregulation of HMGCR occurs in the liver [167], but to our knowledge similar mechanisms have not been reported in the brain. Studies showed high levels of the HMGCR mRNA in all areas of the brain but no obvious differences were found between AD and controls [168]; similarly levels and gene expression of HMGCR were comparable in AD and control samples in another study [169].

FPPS is the last enzyme of the pre-squalene pathway. In two small samples, polymorphisms of FPPS or their haplotypes were associated with AD [8]. But in other samples FPPS variants were not related to AD risk. The AlzGene meta- analysis for FPPS polymorphisms is negative [7].

3.3. Post-squalene pathway

The post-squalene mevalonate pathway is depicted in Figure 4. FPP is converted to squalene by the action of squalene synthase (farnesyl diphosphate farnesyl transferase 1) [170]. Squalene synthase is the first enzyme in the mevalonate pathway whose product, squalene, is committed to cholesterol synthesis. The lack of reports indicating genetic disorders linked to mutations in squalene synthase suggest that this enzyme may be essential in embryonic development (discussed in [114]). In fact, deletion of squalene synthase is embryonic lethal in mice [171]. Squalene synthase is inhibited by zaragozic acid.

Squalene is converted to monooxidosqualene (MOS), which can be further converted to lanosterol and dioxidosqualene (DOS). Formation of both MOS and DOS requires the action of the enzyme squalene monooxygenase (SM) (also called squalene epoxidase). Lanosterol is

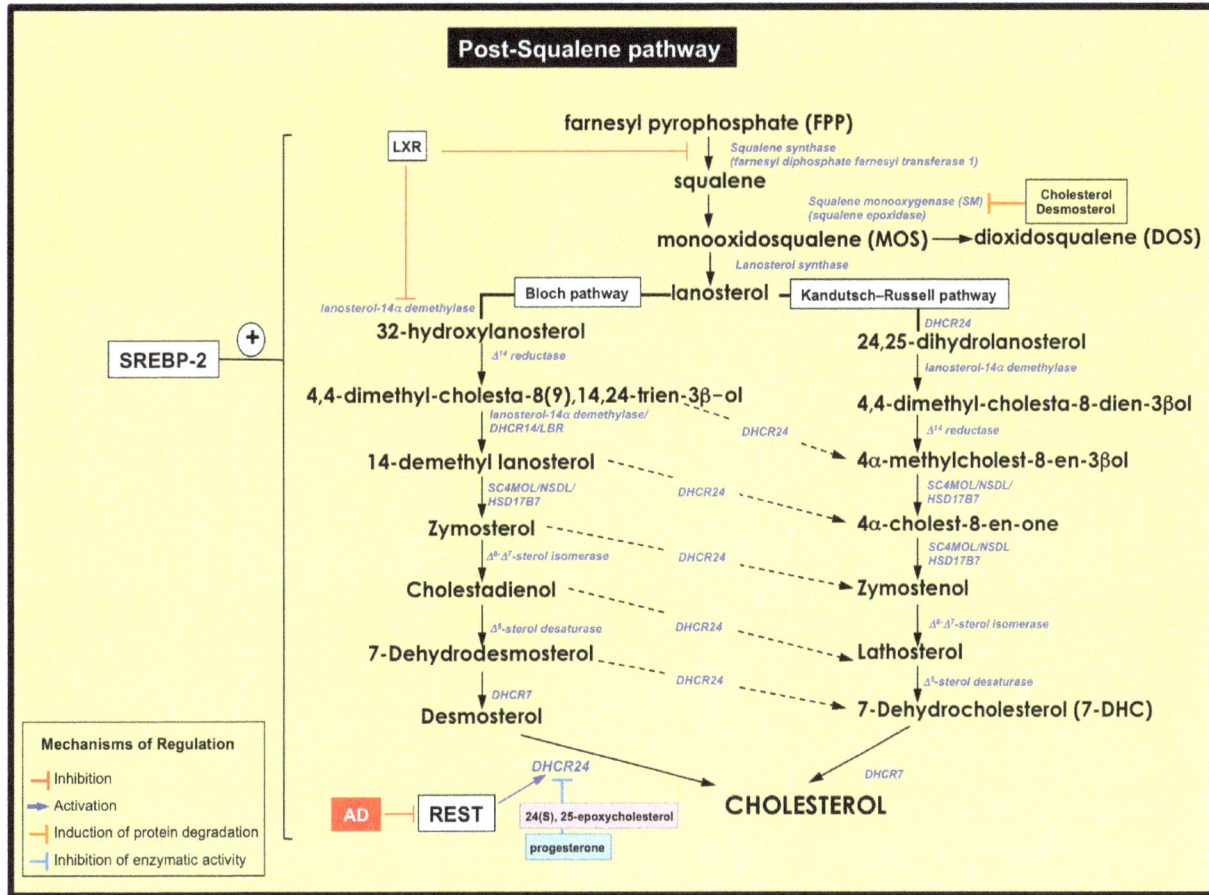

Figure 4. The post-squalene pathway. The final product of the post squalene pathway is cholesterol. Most enzymes of the post-squalene pathway are targets of SREBP-2. Other posttrancriptional regulatory mechanisms also exist.

the first sterol intermediate in cholesterol synthesis. Lanosterol is metabolized to cholesterol by 19 enzymatic steps. In the brain, as in the liver, there are two major pathways for the conversion of lanosterol to cholesterol. The Kandutsch–Russell pathway includes lathosterol and 7-dehydrocholesterol (7-DHC) as intermediates; while the Bloch pathway, uses desmosterol as an intermediate (reviewed in [172]. Post lanosterol precursors are present in all cells that synthesize cholesterol, although they might represent a minor sterol component due to their rapid conversion to downstream metabolites, or to their release from cells [173, 174]. A special scenario is present in embryonic mouse astrocytes, which, freshly dissociated from the striatum or after being cultured for several days, contain desmosterol as a major membrane sterol, accounting for roughly 50% of total sterols [175]. In young rodents, brain cholesterol is mainly synthesized via the desmosterol pathway, while the Kandutsch–Russell pathway is predominant in older rodents [176, 177]. Desmosterol transiently accumulates up to 30% of total sterols in the mammalian brain during development and in the perinatal period indicating the activity of the Bloch pathway [178-183]. In humans the Bloch-pathway plays a minor role in the formation of CNS cholesterol during aging [22]. Neurons and glia seem to use different pathways downstream of lanosterol. Neurons contain precursors for the Kandutsch-Russel pathway (*e.g.*, 7-DHC) whereas astrocytes contain precursors for the Bloch pathway (e.g., desmosterol) [25]. Disturbances in either of these two pathways may result in replacement of cholesterol with its precursors in the brain, which causes serious disorders of the nervous system [184, 185]. Serum lathosterol is considered an indicator of whole body cholesterol synthesis in humans [22, 186, 187]. Lanosterol and desmosterol together with lathosterol are regarded as tissue markers of local cholesterol synthesis [22].

7-DHC and desmosterol are the immediate cholesterol precursors of the Kandutsch-Russel and the Bloch pathways respectively. 7-DHC is converted to cholesterol by 7-DHC reductase (DHCR7). Mutations in the DHCR7 gene cause the human genetic disease Smith-Lemli-Opitz syndrome, characterized by a wide spectrum of developmental anomalies that may result from decreased cholesterol, increased 7-DHC, or a combination of both [184, 188, 189]. Desmosterol is reduced to cholesterol by the enzyme DHCR24, also known as seladin-1 [190]. DHCR24 catalyzes the 24,25-reduction reactions in the cholesterol biosynthesis pathway and may act on most intermediates of the Bloch pathway [23, 114, 191, 192]. Disruption of the DHCR24 gene results in accumulation of desmosterol and is characterized by multiple congenital anomalies in humans and mice [190, 193, 194]. Desmosterol is an abundant structural membrane component in astrocytes [175]. In the brain, high desmosterol levels are present during development [181, 182]. During aging, hippocampal levels of desmosterol decrease significantly in the rat [176]. Desmosterol is a natural ligand of LXR [195].

From the two reductases that participate in the later steps of cholesterol synthesis production, DHCR24 is important in AD and therefore is discussed here in more detail. DHCR24 is encoded by a single gene (Dhcr24) on chromosome 1, an evolutionarily conserved gene with homologies to a family of flavin adenine dinucleotide-dependent oxidoreductases [196]. DHCR24 is detected in many tissues, including brain, adrenal glands, pituitary, thyroid gland, ovary, testis, and prostate [197-199]. Dhcr24 was initially identified as a gene down-regulated in affected brain regions in AD [196] and consequently its product has also been called Seladin-1 from **Se**lective **A**lzheimer's **d**isease **in**dicator 1. However, current evidence indicates that DHCR24 has functions that go beyond those expected from its enzymatic activity in the mevalonate pathway. The roles of DHCR24 in oxidative stress, hepatitis C virus infection, cardiovascular disease, prostate cancer and other conditions have been recently discussed in detail [200]. The role of DHCR24 in AD is discussed in Section 3.3.3.

3.3.1. Shunt in the post-squalene pathway

Conversion of MOS to DOS establishes an alternate pathway leading to the production of (24S, 25)-epoxycholesterol (25-EC) [201] (Figure 2). This shunt in the mevalonate pathway functions in parallel to the conversion of lanosterol to cholesterol [202]. 25-EC is the only oxysterol that does not derive from cholesterol. It is present in rodent brain [203], where it is proportionally more important than 24-HC during development and the perinatal period, but not in the adult [204]. Production of 25-EC represents a cellular defense mechanism against accumulation of cholesterol that derives from the mevalonate pathway (as opposed to exogenously-derived cholesterol) [202]. 25-EC is responsible of the fine-tuning of cholesterol synthesis, and without it, acute cholesterol synthesis is exaggerated [205]. 25-EC is synthesized in both human neurons and astrocytes, and the proportion synthesized by astrocytes is an order of magnitude higher than that of neurons [206]. Astrocytes but not neurons secrete 25-EC and neurons internalize this oxysterol. Interestingly, 25-EC reduced the expression of SREBP-2 target genes and increased expression of LXR target genes in both astrocytes and neurons [205-208]. 25-EC may represent an additional regulatory signal between astrocytes and neurons in cholesterol homeostasis [206]. 25-EC is an important negative regulator of the mevalonate pathway (Section 3.2.1).

3.3.2. Regulation of enzymes of post-squalene pathway

All the enzymes of the post-squalene pathway are transcriptionally activated by SREBP-2 [67, 132, 209]. In addition, LXRα represses transcription of squalene synthase and lanosterol-14α demethylase directly [102].

Posttranslationally, cholesterol and desmosterol but none of the oxysterols enhance SM degradation [210]. MARCH6, also known as Teb4, functions as a selective ubiquitin ligase for SM ubiquitination and consequent proteasomal degradation [146, 211]. Cholesterol-induced degradation of SM is a novel feedback mechanism regulating the mevalonate pathway to prevent cholesterol accumulation without affecting isoprenoid supply.

DHCR24 is regulated by diverse mechanisms at the transcriptional and posttranslational levels. Several studies have identified the Dhcr24 gene as a target of SREBPs [67, 212-214]. In brains of statin-treated mice, there is activation of SREBP-2 and significant up-regulation of DHCR24 in cortex and hippocampus [215]. SREBP-2 binds to two (SREs) present within the Dhcr24 promoter, inducing a novel mode of transcriptional regulation for SREBP-2, characterized by homotypic cooperativity [77]. This type of regulation may warrant that a threshold of active SREBP-2 is reached before committing to the energetically expensive process of cholesterol synthesis [77, 200]. A novel mechanism of DHCR24 transcriptional activation by the transcription factor RE1-silencing transcription factor (REST), which is normally a repressor, has been recently reported [183]. Although this may be a secondary mechanism of DHCR24, the reduced levels of REST present in the brain during development may explain, at least in part, the reduced activity of DHCR24 and the consequent elevation of desmosterol [183]. Interestingly LXR has also been implicated in the regulation of DHCR24 as data from a whole genome screen for LXR binding sites showed that the Dhcr24 gene contained a functional LXR response element [216]. LXR regulation of DHCR24 seems to be tissue specific. LXR did not influence DHCR24 expression in some studies [77], and at least in studies using mice deficient in LXRβ, this regulation does not seem to take place in brain [216]. DHCR24 displays epigenetic regulation by methylation and histone acetylation due to the presence of GC rich regions within the DHCR24 promoter [217]. At the post-translational level DHCR24 activity is inhibited by certain oxysterols (25EC) [218] and by progesterone possibly by direct enzyme inhibition [182]. In addition, a novel mode of DHCR24 inhibition through phosphorylation has been demonstrated, which may allow a rapid inhibition of cholesterol synthesis [219].

3.3.3. Post-squalene pathway in AD

From the enzymes involved in the post-squalene section of the mevalonate pathway, DHCR24 is the most important in AD. A study comparing gene expression by using mRNA differential display identified the down-regulation of DHCR24 in large pyramidal neurons in vulnerable regions in AD but not in healthy brains [196]. This finding was confirmed by others [220], although this may not apply to all AD patients [221]. The down-regulation in DHCR24 transcription was associated with hyperphosphorylated tau but not with β-amyloid deposition [220]. Single nucleotide polymorphisms of DHCR24 have been associated with AD risk [222]. However, these associations have not been confirmed, and other polymorphisms of DHCR24 only associated with AD in men but not in women [223]. Based on the evidence that DHCR24 expression is higher in neural stem cells than in differentiated neurons [224] it was hypothesized that reduced DHCR24 expression might be due to the existence of an impaired neuronal stem cell compartment [225]. Alternatively, transcriptional regulation of DHCR24 may be altered in AD. Indeed, recent studies indicated that the transcription factor REST, identified as a DHCR24 transcriptional activator [183] is lost in mild cognitive impairment and AD [226]. In addition, we have demonstrated that Aβ causes a significant decrease of SREBP-2 activation in neurons [106]; and we found reduced SREBP-2 activation in brain cortex of the AD mouse model CRND8 [107]. These observations suggest that, as the disease progresses reduced DHCR24 levels would not be unique, and that other enzymes of the mevalonate pathway would also be affected in brain cells that accumulate Aβ. However, taking in consideration the cooperative transcriptional mechanism of regulation exerted by SREBP-2 on DHCR24 [77], it is expected that DHCR24 would be particularly sensitive to reduced SREBP-2 activation. A general reduction of the mevalonate pathway could also explain why the levels of desmosterol are decreased in AD brains [227], contrary to what would be predicted if only DHCR24 were down-regulated. If these mechanisms exist in vivo in the brain, then the decrease of DHCR24 would be a consequence, rather than a cause of AD. Contrary to the findings in humans, the levels of desmosterol were elevated in the APPSLxPS1mut mouse model of AD, which also showed a significant decrease in DHCR24 in those brain areas [161]. DHCR24 has neuroprotective effects against Aβ toxicity, ER stress and oxidative stress-induced apoptosis, inhibiting caspase 3 activity and directly scavenging reactive oxygen species [196, 228, 229]. Many other studies have reported the antioxidant properties of DHCR24 in a variety of tissues and in the context of different diseases (reviewed in [200]). Importantly, DHCR24 mediates the protective effects of estrogens in cultured human neuroblasts since estrogen and selective estrogen receptor modulators (SERMs) stimulate the expression of DHCR24 in human neuroblast long-term cell cultures [230, 231]. The neuroprotective action of DHCR24 against Aβ may be due to its ability to maintain plasma membrane cholesterol at levels that prevent the rise of intracellular calcium and the production of ROS and lipoperoxidation that contributes to Aβ toxicity [232-234]. The relevance of these mechanisms in vivo in the brain requires confirmation, especially because there is ample evidence suggesting that high plasma membrane cholesterol may be detrimental in Aβ-induced toxicity (reviewed in [11]). The reduction of cholesterol in cell membranes due to DHCR24 may impair lipid raft functions and favor Aβ accumulation by a combination of inefficient Aβ degradation (due to low plasmin activity) and increased APP amyloidogenic cleavage [235]. Thus, all these mechanisms suggest the existence of vicious feedback cycles involving Aβ and DHCR24.

The post-squalene pathway results in production of cholesterol. There is little consensus about total brain cholesterol alterations in patients with AD [236-238]. Using different methods for measuring cholesterol (discussed in [237]), some studies found no change in cholesterol content in any portion of the brain [239, 240] or the hippocampus [241] in AD brains, while other studies reported changes in cholesterol levels in specific brain areas, particularly in regions with extensive Aβ deposits and neurofibrillary tangles (NFTs). Xiong and collaborators found an increase in cholesterol in the cortex of AD brains [104], Heverin et al. described a significant increase of cholesterol concentration in the basal ganglia but not in other brain areas in a small group of AD brains [242] and Cutler at al. reported accumulation of free cholesterol in the middle frontal gyrus and frontal cortex but not the unaffected cerebellum in AD brains from individuals expressing apoE4 [243]. It was also indicated that, as the severity of the disease progressed, there was an increase in membrane- and amyloid plaque-associated cholesterol [243-245]. Cholesterol levels were lower in the temporal gyrus of autopsied brains of AD patients compared to control subjects [246].

Analysis of post squalene cholesterol precursors also provided conflicting results. Lathosterol was reported to be elevated in the basal ganglia and the pons in AD but the ratio of lathosterol to cholesterol, used as a marker for cholesterol synthesis, was not significantly different between controls and AD patients suggesting that cholesterol synthesis is normal [242]. More recently a model for cholesterol homeostasis deregulation was proposed based on the measurement of post-squalene cholesterol precursors, cholesterol and oxysterol in brains of individuals with no-cognitive impairment, MCI and AD [247]. In 'compensated' MCI and initial AD there would be a heme oxygenase-1-mediated stimulation of cholesterol synthesis and cholesterol efflux in the astroglial compartment to allow cholesterol delivery for neuronal repair. As the disease progresses, massive uptake of cholesterol derived from widespread neuronal degeneration would overwhelm glial efflux pathways resulting in increased brain cholesterol levels and feed-back suppression of de novo cholesterol synthesis. This model could explain the findings in CSF. In CSF, cholesterol levels were significantly lower in AD patients as compared to controls [248, 249], and absolute levels of lanosterol, lathosterol and desmosterol and ratios of cholesterol precursors/cholesterol were also significantly reduced strongly indicating that *de novo* cholesterol synthesis within the CNS of AD patients might be impaired [248]. In the latter study, only the ratio of desmosterol/cholesterol was not significantly different in AD patients as compared to controls, but the increased CSF ratios of desmosterol/lathosterol suggests that the activity of the Kandutsch–Russell pathway might be reduced more than the Bloch pathway. The authors proposed that reduced expression of DHCR24 also contributes to decreased levels of cholesterol in AD patients and may explain the high levels of desmosterol found in AD in some studies [220, 250]. However, in other cases brain levels of desmosterol were reduced in AD [227]. This last finding agrees with the possibility that mevalonate pathway enzymes other than DHCR24 may also be down-regulated in AD, perhaps by a mechanism that involves SREBP-2 inhibititon. A further indication that cholesterol synthesis might be inhibited in AD is the finding that neurosteroids, which result from cholesterol metabolism, are reduced in AD temporal cortex as compared to control subjects [251]. It is important to highlight that changes in levels of cholesterol intermediates in brains of mouse AD models do not parallel changes in human patients. In the APP transgenic mice carrying the Swedish mutation (APP23), no differences in the levels of lathosterol, desmosterol or cholesterol and were found when compared with wild-type animals [177]. These differences must be considered when using animal models to study the mevalonate pathway.

It is possible that a change in the distribution of cholesterol inside brain cells rather than a change in total cholesterol content may influence AD pathology [252]. We have shown that Aβ induces cholesterol sequestration within the neuronal endosomal/lysosomal system, and impairs intracellular trafficking [106]. Our findings provide an explanation to the cellular cholesterol overload reported in brains of AD patients [253]. They also agree with previous work that showed cholesterol sequestration specifically in Aβ-immunopositive neurons [104, 254, 255], and with studies in transgenic mouse models of AD where cholesterol sequestration in the brain was preceded by Aβ accumulation and/or coincided with areas of Aβ accumulation [244, 256, 257]. These studies underscored the relevance of cholesterol sequestration in AD. This is important because a causal relationship between cellular cholesterol sequestration and cell death has been found in Niemann-Pick Type C (NPC) pathology [258]. NPC is a disorder characterized by impairment of intracellular cholesterol trafficking and cholesterol sequestration in the endosomal compartment [259]. Accumulation of cholesterol within the endosomal-lysosomal system in NPC not only triggers degeneration of neurons in selected brain regions but also leads to abnormal processing of APP and Aβ generation as observed in AD pathology. The similarities between AD and NPC include the presence of immunologically similar tau-positive NFTs [254, 260], the influence of ε4 isoform of apoE in promoting disease pathology [261], and endosomal abnormalities associated with the accumulation of cleaved APP derivatives and/or Aβ peptides in vulnerable neurons [262, 263]. Importantly, strategies previously used to reduce cholesterol sequestration in NPC and strategies that reduce cholesterol levels by increasing cholesterol metabolism improved pathological symptoms in mouse models of AD [264, 265].

Preclinical and clinical studies have indicated the critical role of cholesterol in AD. This topic has been reviewed extensively and thoroughly in the past years [11, 12, 18, 236, 238, 266-268], thus it is not discussed in this chapter. The best-studied role of cholesterol is in the production of Aβ from amyloid precursor protein (APP). Overall, the evidence indicates that increase in cellular cholesterol causes an increase in Aβ production, although some studies showed the opposite [11, 12, 269]. Cholesterol regulates Aβ uptake and toxicity, but the evidence on whether cholesterol reduces or favors Aβ toxicity is controversial [11, 12]. Brain cholesterol is important in synapse development and maintenance [27, 270, 271]. Synaptic dysfunction is one of the earliest significant events in AD and synapse loss is the strongest anatomical correlate of the degree of clinical impairment [272, 273]. Significant decrease in dendritic spine density is present in the hippocampus of patients with AD and in transgenic mouse models of AD [274-278]. Alterations in cholesterol levels, even locally at synapses, may play a role in synapse dysfunction in AD [279].

3.4. Non-sterol isoprenoids pathway

The branch of the mevalonate pathway that leads to the production of non-sterol isoprenoids is depicted in Figure 5. The enzymes involved in these steps have been extensively reviewed [59]. The importance of this pathway is emphasized by the number of diseases that are associated with its dysfunction, including AD, Parkinson's disease, cancer, and tuberculosis [129, 280-282].

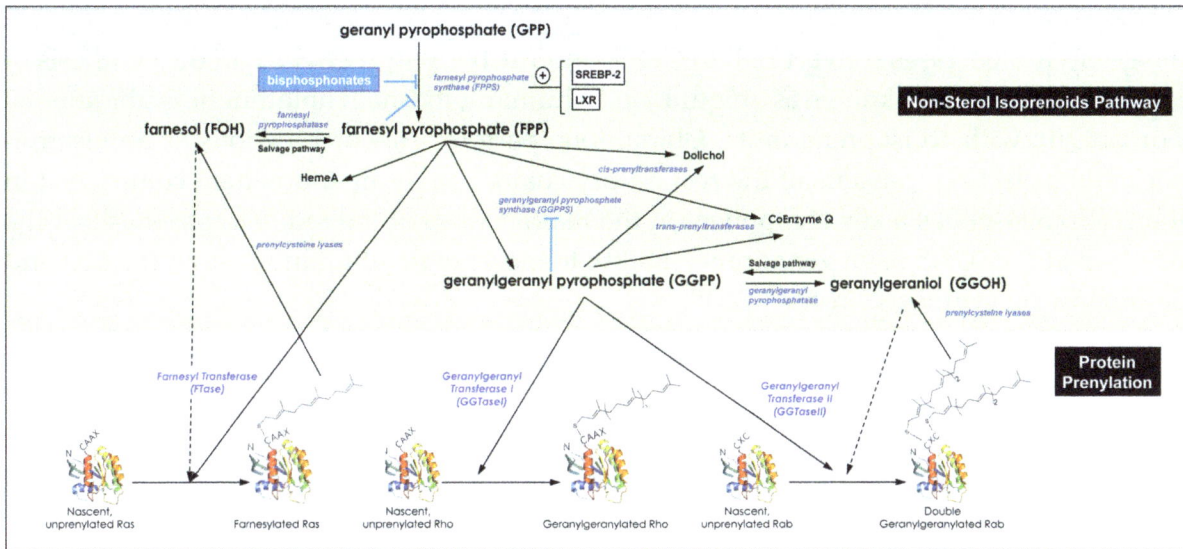

Figure 5. The non-sterol isoprenoid pathway.

FPP is the common substrate for synthesis of several end products and for the lipid modification of proteins. The enzymes responsible for synthesis of FPP and its non-sterol derivatives are prenyl-transferases that catalyze consecutive condensations of IPPs with primer substrates to form linear backbones for all isoprenoid compounds [130]. The enzyme GGPPS catalyzes the conversion of FPP into GGPP [283]. The main role of FPP and GGPP is in the posttranslational isoprenylation (*i.e.* farnesylation and geranylgeranylation) of proteins (Section 3.4.1.). Two different GGPPS activities have been described: a membrane-associated protein that produces GGPP for dolichol biosynthesis and a cytosolic protein that produces GGPP for protein prenylation [284]. In mouse brain cytosol, FPPS and GGPPS activities were higher than those in the corresponding fractions from the liver, perhaps reflecting a higher demand for protein prenylation in the brain [284]. FPPS and GGPPS activities were differentially distributed across various subregions of the brain. FPPS activity was present in all brain regions as expected by the several products that derive from FPP [285]. GGPPS activity was ~100 fold lower than FPPS activity, which agrees with the more limited use of GGPP, mostly for protein prenylation and as a precursor of a limited number of metabolites. GGPPS activity was lowest in the cerebellum [285].There have not been any reported cases of FPPS or GGPPS deficiency in humans [128]. FPPS is the target of nitrogen-containing bisphosphonate (N-BP) inhibitors, drugs used extensively to treat bone diseases [286]. A few bisphosphonate selective inhibitors for GGPPS have been reported but a clinically proven inhibitor of GGPPS has not yet been identified, limiting the validation of this enzyme as a therapeutic target [287].

Cis-prenyltransferases enzymes use FPP and GGPP for synthesis of dolichols [288, 289]. Dolichol phosphate is a lipid carrier embedded in the ER membrane, essential for the synthesis of N-glycans, GPI-anchors and protein C- and O-mannosylation [290, 291]. Dolichol is present, as a family with different chain lengths, in the hippocampus and spinal cord in a relatively low concentration compared to other areas of the brain [285]. Dolichol increases in brain and in peripheral organs during aging [292] and is associated with increased HMGCR activity [293]. The use of dolichol level as a marker for aging has been proposed [294].

Trans-prenyltransferases convert FPP to GGPP and further polyprenyl-PP in the synthesis of Coenzyme Q (CoQ), also known as ubiquinone. In humans, the main ubiquinone is ubiquinone 10, or CoQ10, with 10 isoprene units. Ubiquinone performs major functions as an electron carrier in the electron transfers of the respiratory chain, and as an antioxidant component in cell membranes and as a key component in the maintenance of the redox homeostasis of the cell [295-298]. The CNS has a very limited ability to incorporate ubiquinone from the diet and relies mainly on synthesis "in situ" [299].

FPP and GGPP can be converted to their correspondent alcohols farnesol (FOH) and geranyl-geranyol (GGOH) by farnesyl and geranylgeranyl pyrophosphatases [300, 301]. Salvage pathways for the conversion of FOH and GGOH back to their pyrophosphate counterpart seem to exist in mammalian cells [302]. FOH and GGOH can also be formed by degradation of isoprenylated proteins in reactions catalyzed by prenylcysteine lyases, enzymes highly expressed in the brain [303]. FOH and GGOH may down-regulate HMGCR (Section 3.2.1 and Figure 3) (reviewed in [128]). The role of FOH and GGOH in protein prenylation is unclear. Some studies showed that mammalian cells utilize exogenously supplied FOH and GGOH for protein isoprenylation and, when mevalonate biosynthesis is blocked by statins, free FOH and GGOH can restore the pools of FPP and GGPP, although FOH may not be converted to GGPP [302, 304, 305]. The use of FOH and/or GGOH for protein prenylation might occur preferentially under conditions of reduced FPP and GGPP production from mevalonate [306]. Contrary to the existence of a salvage pathway that uses FOH and GGOH for protein prenylation, it was demonstrated that overexpressing phosphatases that convert FPP and GGPP to FOH and GGOH in mammalian cells, decreases rather than increases protein isoprenylation (as evaluated by a decreased of Rho protein level in cell membranes) and results in defects in cell growth and cytoskeletal organization that are associated with dysregulation of Rho family GTPases [301]. Moreover, work in cancer cells proposed that GGOH would reduce protein prenylation by down-regulating HMGCR leading to a shortage of FPP and GGPP [307]. Whether any of these mechanisms take place in the brain is uncertain. FOH is present at physiologically relevant concentrations in the brain of rodents and humans, where it may act in the regulation of brain Ca^{2+} homeostasis and neurotransmitter release by inhibiting N-type Ca^{2+} channels [308]. FOH has been shown to modulate the activity of the farnesoid X receptor (FXR), a member of the nuclear hormone receptor superfamily [309].

3.4.1. Non-sterol isoprenoids and protein prenylation

FPP and GGPP are substrates for protein farnesylation and geranylgeranylation (collectively called isoprenylation). In the human genome, there are approximately 300 hypothetical prenylated proteins [310]. Among them heterotrimeric G protein subunits, nuclear lamins and small GTPases have been confirmed to be prenylated [311]. Small GTPases represent the largest group of prenylated proteins. All small GTPases are able to specifically bind GDP and GTP, being inactive when bound to GDP (cytosolic location) and active when bound to GTP (membrane location). They also have an intrinsic GTPase activity to hydrolyze bound GTP to GDP and phosphate (Pi) [312]. FPP and GGPP are covalently attached via thioester linkage to C-terminal cysteine residues in the context of a prenylation motif. Farnesylation is catalyzed by farnesyl protein transferase (FTase), whereas GGTase-I and geranylgeranyl transferase type II (GGTase II) or RabGGTase catalyze the addition of GGPP to specific subsets of proteins [313-315] (Figure 5). FTase and GGTase I are responsible for posttranslational lipidation of proteins with C- terminal "CAAX" motifs, where C is cysteine, A is often an aliphatic amino acid, and X at the C-terminus determines the specificity of protein prenylation. When X is a methionine or serine, as in Ras proteins, then the protein is farnesylated by FTase. However, when X is a leucine residue, as in Rho proteins (e.g. Rac1, Cdc42, RhoA), or a phenylalanine residue, then the protein is geranylgeranylated by GGTase I [316, 317]. GGTase II catalyzes prenylation of Rab proteins, which contain at their C-termini either one or, more frequently, two cysteine residues, both of which are modified by geranylgeranyl groups [318, 319]. Protein prenyltransferase inhibitors, namely FTase inhibitors (FTIs) and GGTase inhibitors (GGTIs) have been developed and evaluated as anticancer agents.

The covalent attachment of the lipophilic isoprenyl group(s) enables prenylated proteins to anchor to cell membranes, which is an essential requirement for biological function [311]. The localization of small GTPases in distinct subcellular sites defines which signaling pathways they activate, thus defining their participation in disease. As an example, some singly preny-lated Rabs are mistargeted and dysfunctional [320]. Inhibiting the membrane localization of small GTPases is a therapeutic strategy in cancer [321]. In addition, isoprenoid moieties are essential in the protein-protein interaction functions of prenylated proteins since they work as molecular handles that bind to hydrophobic grooves on the surface of soluble protein factors; these factors remove the prenylated protein from membranes in a regulated manner [322]. There is evidence that unprenylated versions of some proteins may also have physiological functional effects [323, 324] or may interfere with the activity of the isoprenylated proteins during disease [325, 326]. The requirement of prenylation for membrane association has also been recently challenged [327]. Prenylated proteins may undergo other posttranslational modifications such as palmitoylation, miristoylation and/or carboxymethylation [328].

The interest in understanding the regulation of isoprenoid production and protein prenylation in the brain has increased considerably in the past few years due to the importance of protein prenylation in several cellular processes such as cell growth, cytoskeletal organization and remodeling, and vesicle trafficking; and to the fact that some of the beneficial effects of statins in neurodegenerative diseases have been attributed to changes of protein prenylation [129, 329-334]. Non-sterol isoprenoids and protein prenyltransferases have emerged as attractive therapeutic targets for several diseases [321, 329] but we still need a deeper understanding of their roles in the brain in order to determine their value for treating neurodegeneration in general, and AD in particular.

Until recently, protein prenylation was considered to function constitutively. However, there is evidence that signaling cascades activated by druggable surface receptors affect prenylation of specific small GTPases by posttranslational modifications (e.g. phosphorylation) of unprenylated versions of the protein [326], or by regulating protein prenyltransferases directly [335]. Prenyltransferases are expressed in the brain, which contains the highest activity of GGTase I [336]. GGTase I plays important roles in synapse formation, where it is activated through acetylcholine receptor clustering at the postsynaptic membrane [335]. The effects of GGTase I at the synapse were suggested to be due to geranylgeranylation of Rho GTPases, although prenylation was not directly examined. Neuronal depolarization and BDNF activated GGTase I and this activity was required for dendritic arborization in hippocampal neurons and Purkinje cells [337-339].

There is a growing body of evidence indicating that inhibition of protein prenyltransferases and inhibition of the mevalonate pathway to an extent that reduces the levels of FPP and GGPP, alter many mechanisms critical for normal brain function. When analyzing studies in which statins are used it is important to consider that different statins differ in terms of their potency, stability and ability to cross the BBB [329, 331, 340]. Studies on the effect of statins or protein prenyl transferase inhibitors on neurite (dendrites or axons) extension and branching provided conflicting results depending on the type of neurons, the class of statin used and the duration of the treatments. Some studies showed that statins or inhibitors of protein prenyltransferases enhanced neurite outgrowth, number, length and/or branching [341-344] while we and others, discovered inhibition of neurite outgrowth, extension or branching [345-347]. Statins decreased neurite initiation but increased neurite branching in neuroblastoma cells [348]. The field of AD research will benefit from a deeper understanding of the roles of non-sterol isoprenoids and protein prenylation in axon regrowth.

Under certain experimental conditions statins affect survival of neurons and neuron-like cells, acting through the decrease of non-sterol isoprenoids and protein prenylation. Lovastatin but not pravastatin induced apoptosis of rat brain neuroblasts and caused a significant reduction of the membrane pool of Ras and RhoA proteins, suggesting an impairment of protein prenylation as the result of reduced isoprenoid production [349]. Similarly, we found no effect of pravastatin on survival of sympathetic and cortical neurons at concentrations that significantly reduced cholesterol synthesis [106, 347, 350]. Under these conditions, however, pravastatin did not affect protein prenylation [106]. Statins induced stellation, followed by apoptosis in cerebellar astrocytes and cell death of cerebellar neurons [351]. These latter effects were independent of reduced cholesterol synthesis but were prevented by GGPP. A very interesting discovery from the work of Marz and colleagues [351] was that neuronal cell death was significantly reduced in astrocyte/neuron co-cultures treated with statins. The authors speculated that astroglia cells might provide neuroprotective signals, perhaps GGPP, against the damaging effects that result from downregulation the mevalonate pathway. This idea of communication between glia and neurons through intermediates of the mevalonate pathway is further discussed in Section 4.

Non-sterol isoprenoids and protein prenylation may play a role in inflammatory events in the brain since statins were able to activate microglia in cultured rat hippocampal slices [352], and inhibitors of protein prenyltransferases and statins caused a reduction of apoE secretion by cultured microglia and organotypic hippocampal cultures [353]. Contradictory evidence was reported on the role of non-sterol isoprenoids and protein prenylation in long-term potentiation (LTP), an experimental model to study the synaptic basis of learning and memory [354]. While inhibitors of FTase and GGTase I had no effects on LTP in one study [355], FPP depletion and farnesylation inhibition were implicated in the enhancement of the LTP magnitude in hippocampal slices [356].

In the majority of the studies the conclusion that the effects of statins were due to the reduction of non-sterol isoprenoids and protein prenylation resulted from experiments in which FPP, GGPP or their correspondent alcohols, but not cholesterol were able to prevent the particular effect [343, 345, 346, 348, 352, 353, 357]. It will be important however, to confirm that protein prenylation is impaired upon statin treatment, especially when the duration of the treatment is short such as in the studies by Mans et al. [356]. Different prenylated proteins have half-lives that vary between 4hs and 24hs and will be differentially affected. The time required for depletion of the non-sterol isoprenoids pools may also be tissue-or cell-specific. Only a few studies examined the effect of statins on protein prenylation directly and found decreased prenylation of specific proteins under specific experimental conditions [341, 346].

The Rho family of GTPases has received a lot of attention as the mediators of the effects that result from reduction of non-sterol isoprenoids and/or inhibition of protein prenyl transferases [335, 337, 338, 341, 346, 352, 358]. This family represents a major branch of the Ras superfamily, and like Ras and Rabs, Rho proteins (e.g., RhoA, Rac1, Cdc42) function as GTP/GDP switches and alternate between an active GTP-bound state and an inactive GDP-bound state. Members of the Rho family are farnersylated and/or geranylgeranylated through the action of GGTase I [359]. Rho GTPases are pivotal in the integration of extracellular and intracellular signals. They are key regulators of the actin cytoskeleton which plays essential roles in orchestrating the development and remodeling of spines and synapses [360, 361]. Precise spatio-temporal regulation of Rho GTPase activity is critical for their function. Aberrant Rho GTPase signaling due to mutations or other causes can cause spine and synapse defects resulting in abnormal neuronal connectivity and deficient cognitive functioning in humans [360, 361]. Recent findings indicate that Rho GTPases are key components of neuronal cell degeneration pathways [362]. A number of studies examined the localization of Rho proteins to the membranes as an indication of their prenylation status. A caveat of this approach is that some prenylated Rho proteins interact with the guanidine dissociation inhibitor RhoGDI, which keep prenylated Rho proteins in the cytosol in an inactive state [363]. RhoGDI expression is affected during disease [363]. A decreased in RhoA or Rac association with membranes has been observed upon treatment with statins or protein prenyltransferase inhibitors [337, 338, 341, 346, 352]. A decrease in GTP-bound forms of Rho family proteins was also detected upon statin or protein prenyltransferase inhibitor treatments [338, 343] Moreover, RhoA was identified as a modulator of statins effects by using an unbiased genome-wide filter approach that examine more than 10,000 genes to identify gene expression changes that correlated with altered expression of HMGCR [364].

Non-sterol isoprenoids and protein prenylation not only determine the targeting of prenylated proteins to membranes, but also regulate the expression of a subset of prenylated proteins in a protein-specific manner [365, 366]. Depletion of mevalonate or treatment with protein prenyltransferase inhibitors resulted in up-regulation of Ras, Rac1, RhoB, Rab5 and Rab7 [365, 367-369]. The increase occurs at the levels of mRNA and protein in most cases, and both unprenylated and isoprenylated forms of the proteins accumulate [365]. Reduction of non-sterol isoprenoids decreases protein degradation, including that of already isoprenylated proteins, which suggests the existence of regulatory mechanisms to sustain levels of isoprenylated proteins under conditions that would otherwise limit protein isoprenylation [370]. FPP or GGPP prevented protein up-regulation [367, 370] by transcriptional and posttranscriptional mechanisms still unidentified but independent of protein prenylation [370]. In the case of Rab proteins it has been proposed that the membrane pool of Rabs, which decreases upon depletion of GGPP, may serve as an intracellular signal for Rab expression regulation [369].

3.4.2. Regulation of enzymes of non-sterol isoprenoids pathway

FPPS is transcriptionally regulated by SREBP-2 [66, 371] and LXR [372]. A LXR response element sequence exists in the FPPS promoter overlapping with the SREBP-2 response element [372]. LXR activation of FPPS occurs under high cholesterol levels, thus SREBP-2 processing is inhibited. In this way LXR could drive the expression of FPPS in order to maintain isoprenoid supply exclusively [372]. FPPS is post-translationally regulated by a product-feedback competitive inhibition as FPP (product) competes with GPP (substrate) for the active site [373, 374].

GGPPS does not seem to be transcriptionally regulated by SREBP-2 [66, 284, 375, 376]. GGPPS activity is inhibited by GGPP [373]. The crystal structure of human GGPPS demonstrated GGPP binding to a pocket/cavity away from the chain elongation site (active site) of GGPPS, suggesting a product-feedback allosteric inhibition [377, 378]. Mammalian GGPPS can catalyze the formation of FPP as well as GGPP [379].

3.4.3. Coordination of the post-squalene and non-sterol isoprenoids branches of the mevalonate pathway

Since cells have two alternative sources of cholesterol namely intracellular synthesis and uptake but only the intracellular synthesis provides non-sterol isoprenoids, the mevalonate pathway has to maintain the minimum requirement of isoprenoids at all times irrespective of cholesterol levels. Analysis of the affinity of the enzymes in the different branches of the pathway uncovers the mechanisms that mediate such regulation. The affinity of GGPPS for FPP (K_m value of 0.6 μM) [284] is much higher than the affinity of squalene synthase for FPP (Km value of ~15 μM) [380]. Moreover, both coenzyme Q and dolichol synthesis are saturated at a much lower concentration of isoprene intermediates than the concentration required to saturate cholesterol synthesis [381, 382]. Thus, under limited concentrations of mevalonate and FPP, the non-sterol isoprenoid branch will be favored. Furthermore, inhibition of the mevalonate production by statins will reduce FPP supply for the production of cholesterol first. Because of the very high affinity of protein farnesyl transferase for FPP (Km below 0.1 μM) [383], farnesylation is preserved under many statin treatments [297, 384] and would be favored over geranylgeranylation.

3.4.4. Non-sterol isoprenoid pathway in AD

Up-regulation of 6 out of 10 genes of isoprenoid metabolism was found in autopsied hippocampus of patients with incipient AD [105], which may represent an attempt to compensate the posttranslational inhibition of the mevalonate pathway during disease.

Dolichol is decreased in all areas of the AD brain, especially those regions affected by the disease, and dolichol-P increases in brain regions that showed morphological changes [239, 385]. In the frontal cortex and in the hippocampus the concentration of dolichol decreased by as much as 45%. The increase in dolichol-P may reflect an increased rate of glycosylation in AD brain, which may be related to the formation of amyloid plaques. Changes in dolichol and dolichol-P in AD are opposite to those present during normal aging. The amount of dolichol in different regions of the human brain, but especially in the hippocampus, increases several folds with age in humans [239, 292, 386] and rats [387, 388]. An upper limit for dolichol accumulation in tissues seems to exist since after 70 years of age there is no further increase in dolichol concentration in human brains [239]. Dolichol is present in the brain as a family with 17-21 isoprene units. This pattern of dolichol lengths is unchanged during aging; however, there are regional differences [239, 386]. Levels of dolichyl-P are already high at the time of birth and only show a moderate increase, although it varies between different brain regions [292, 386].

With respect to ubiquinone, there is a significant elevation in most regions of AD brain [239], which may reflect a futile attempt to protect the brain from oxidative stress [385]. Interestingly, the pattern of ubiquinone is also reversed in AD when compared with normal aging. Brain ubiquinone is unchanged up to the age of 55 but decreases significantly in older age groups in areas where it concentrates in human brains, mainly the nucleus caudatus, gray matter, and hippocampus [239, 386]. This decrease may indicate a reduced anti-oxidative capacity in the aging brain. Thus, when considering dolichol, dolichol-P and ubiquinone, AD cannot be regarded as a result of premature aging.

3.4.5. FPP, GGPP and protein prenylation in AD

There is limited information with respect to levels and regulation of FPP and GGPP in normal and AD brains. Recent studies showed that GGPP, FPP, and the mRNA of their respective synthases, FPPS and GGPPS, were elevated in brains of 13 male patients with AD [169], in brains of aged mice [129, 287] and in neuroblastoma SH-SY5Y cells expressing APP695 [389]. The significance of this elevation is still unknown because protein prenylation was not examined in these studies, and elevation of isoprenoids does not warrant an increase in protein prenylation. Indeed, even when GGPP levels were elevated in the aging mouse brain, the pools of Rac1, RhoA and Cdc42, associated to membranes were decreased, while Rab proteins had a mixed behavior [287]. The reduction of the subunit β of GGTase I in the aging brain may be responsible for the decreased prenylation.

The roles of non-sterol isoprenoids and protein prenylation in AD have been identified mainly by using statins and inhibitors of protein prenyltransferases. FPP, GGPP and prenylated proteins are involved in diverse processes important in AD pathology including APP metabolism, LTP and synaptic plasticity, Aβ toxicity, and oxidative stress.

The effects of statin-induced non-sterol isoprenoids depletion or inhibition of protein prenyltransferases on APP/Aβ metabolism are complex. In some cases treatment with statins or a FTase inhibitor stimulated the shedding of APP and the production of sAPPα in neuroblastoma cells overexpressing APPswe [390], while in other cases statins reduced the release of

Aβ from cells but increased the intracellular accumulation of APP and Aβ, in a process prevented by GGPP [391, 392]. The proteins affected by shortage of non-sterol isoprenoids, and responsible for the regulation APP/Aβ metabolism have been identified or proposed. The increase in APP shedding was mediated by RHO proteins [390]. Rho was also suggested to be responsible for the reduction of brain Aβ levels in the AD CRND8 mouse treated with statins, although there was no direct evidence that isoprenylation was affected [393]. The accumulation of APP and Aβ within neurons that received statins was due to decreased delivery of Rab proteins to cell membranes [392]. It is known that Rabs participate in intracellular APP trafficking and processing [394]. A study of mice treated with statins has shown significant reduction of brain levels of Aβ and the C-terminal fragments (CTFs) due to enhanced trafficking of APP-CTFs to the lysosomes for degradation [395]. The authors suggested that the process may involve a decrease in isoprenoids, and would be mediated by Rabs. However, Rab prenylation was not measured in this study and the conclusion of the involvement of isoprenoids resulted from experiments in cultured neurons in which mevalonate prevented the changes in trafficking. Unless the concentration of mevalonate is titrated to recover specifically the non-sterol isoprenoid pathway, mevalonate would also affect cholesterol levels. The regulation of APP cleavage and Aβ production by non-sterol isoprenoids and protein prenylation also involved APP secretases, although it is unclear if the decrease or the increase in isoprenoids and protein prenylation favors amyloidogenic processing of APP. Inhibition of farnesylation reduced the association of the β-secretase enzyme BACE1 with APP (although BACE itself is not farnesylated) and resulted in a dose-dependent decrease in Aβ release and production within the cell [396]. Moreover, statins caused inhibition of β-secretase dimerization into its more active form, which may be a mechanism of the reduction in Aβ production [397]. Statins also significantly decreased the association of the γ-secretase complex with lipid rafts and GGOH prevented this [398]. Contrary to this notion, in a separate study statins induced an increase of BACE levels in neurons, which was linked to the increase in Aβ production [391]. GGOH, GGPP and FPP increased Aβ production by targeting γ-secretase [399-401] but there is no consensus if this effect is dependent [401] or independent [400] of protein prenylation.

Aβ production is not significantly altered in sporadic forms of AD, which represent approximately 95% of cases [402-404]. Instead, defects in Aβ removal may be key in the development of sporadic AD [405, 406]. Statins and an FTase inhibitor promoted degradation of extracellular Aβ by microglia by stimulating the secretion of IDE (insulin degrading enzyme), an enzyme that degrades Aβ in the brain [407]. The secretion of IDE from peripheral organs into the circulation was also increased in mice treated with statins [407]. Moreover FTase but not GGTase I haplodeficiency in the APPPS1 mice increased steady-state levels of IDE [408]. The mechanisms by which farnesylation may regulate IDE secretion, are still unclear.

We have discovered that in neurons challenged with oligomeric Aβ$_{42}$, and in the cortex of the AD mouse CRND8, prenylation of Rabs and Ras proteins were reduced [106]. Since the deficit in protein prenylation induced by Aβ was prevented by GGPP we concluded that protein prenylation inhibition was due to a shortage of GGPP. More importantly GGPP was able to prevent Aβ-induced neuronal death.

Non-sterol isoprenoids have been associated with the regulation of neuroinflammation in AD. The role of inflammation in the AD brain is well known. The pro-inflammatory response mediated mainly by microglial may exacerbate and drive the pathogenic processes leading to neuronal loss. Microglia activation may occur as a response to Aβ accumulation in the brain. Statins inhibited the production of IL-1β by monocytes after stimulation with Aβ, in a process that is independent of cholesterol but prevented by GGPP [409]. The effect was mimicked by a GGTase I inhibitor and by inactivation of Rho proteins. Statins also induced cholesterol-independent inhibition of ROS production after stimulation with Aβ [409]. Statin treatment of microglia resulted in perturbation of the cytoskeleton and morphological changes due to alteration in Rho family function [410].

During the course of AD, tau is hyper-phosphorylated, detaches from the microtubules, and aggregates in the somatodendritic compartment in NFTs [411, 412]. There is very limited information about the existence of any relationship between tau pathology and isoprenoids and/or protein prenylation. Statins caused changes in tau phosphorylation that were characteristic of those observed in preclinical stages of AD [413]. These changes were mimicked by GGTase I inhibitors and compensated by GGPP suggesting that decreased prenylation of a Rho family member may be involved. The dose of statins seems to be critical in the effects on tau. In a cellular model of tauopathy, and in primary neurons, low-to-moderate doses of statins, reduced total and phosphorylated tau levels but high doses activated caspase 3 and increased levels of caspase-cleaved tau, which may facilitate tau Aβ toxicity/apoptosis [414]. A decrease in membrane localization of several small GTPases occurred concomitantly with tau reduction and GGPP reversed statin-induced decreases in tau levels. The authors focused their attention on RhoA, speculating that the statin-induced decrease in phosphorylated tau was caused by glycogen synthase kinase 3β (GSK3β) inactivation through RhoA [414].

Some recent work in genetically modified mice supported the concept that non-sterol isoprenoids and protein prenylation may have a detrimental role in AD and suggested that inhibition of protein prenylation could be a potential strategy for effectively treating AD. The increase of isoprenoids and protein prenylation has been suggested (although not tested) to contribute to tau pathology in a transgenic APP/PS1 mouse that constitutively overexpresses (P)SREBP-2 [415]. In a different mouse model the expression of protein prenyltransferases was genetically modified in order to reduce protein prenylation independent of non-sterol isoprenoids. Heterozygous deletion of FTase reduced Aβ deposition and neuroinflammation and rescued spatial learning and memory function in APPPS1 mice. Heterozygous deletion of GGTase I reduced the levels of Aβ and neuroinflammation but had no impact on learning and memory [408]. These studies in vivo are exciting but will benefit from direct measurement of brain levels of isoprenoids or protein prenylation. Based on the complex regulation of isoprenoid production, it will be important to determine if brain isoprenoid levels change in these mice since the existence of negative-feedback regulatory mechanisms downstream SREBP-2, argue that increased levels of active SREBP-2 does not warrant an increase in non-sterol isoprenoids.

A few prenylated proteins have been linked to AD. The contributions of Rho GTPases to AD are of particular interest. Rho-family GTPases are key proteins that integrate extracellular and intracellular signals. They are important regulators of the actin cytoskeleton that play essential roles in orchestrating the development and remodeling of spines and synapses [360, 361]. Precise spatio-temporal regulation of Rho GTPase activity is critical for their function. Aberrant Rho GTPase signaling due to mutations or other causes can cause spine and synapse defects resulting in abnormal neuronal connectivity and deficient cognitive functioning in humans [360, 361]. Deregulation of RhoGTPases may contribute to dendritic spine loss during AD and might be a key pathogenic event contributing to synaptic deficits in AD (reviewed in [362, 416]). RhoA protein was lower in the AD brain hippocampus, reflecting the loss of the membrane bound, presumably active, GTPase [417]. Rab proteins regulate intracellular membrane trafficking, motility and fusion [418]. In the nervous system Rabs participate in important processes such as axonal endocytosis, retrograde transport of growth signals, synaptic function, and polarized neurite growth [419]. Rab5 and Rab7 protein levels were upregulated within basal forebrain, frontal cortex, and hippocampus but not in the less vulnerable cerebellum and striatum in MCI and AD [420, 421]. Importantly, this upregulation correlated with cognitive decline and neuropathological criteria for AD. The increase of Rab7 and Rab5 in AD brains has been interpreted as overactivation of the endosomal pathway. In addition increased levels of Rab7 have been found in cerebrospinal fluid (CSF) from AD patients and may represent a novel AD CSF biomarker [422]. Evidence from our laboratory demonstrated increased levels of Rab7 in Aβ-treated neurons and in the cortex of CRND8 mice [107]. Rab-6 was increased in AD brain, and correlated with ER stress [423]. The increased level of Rab6 in AD was unable to protect against ER stress, suggesting that Rab6 is non-functional. Based on our discoveries, we anticipate that Rab6 prenylation may be decreased. Since the number of proteins that are prenylated is high and considering that a reduction of non-sterol isoprenoids or the inhibition of protein prenyltransferases will affect several prenylated proteins, the challenge in the next years will be to identify which prenylated proteins are affected in AD.

4. Conclusions

The analysis of the mevalonate pathway in AD reveals dysregulation. The abnormalities not only affect cholesterol but also non-sterol isoprenoids. There is a reciprocal regulation between Aβ and cholesterol at the subcellular level [11]. The evidence discussed here suggest that similar reciprocity may exist between Aβ and non-sterol isoprenoids such that isoprenylation determines the levels of intracellular Aβ [391, 392] and Aβ inhibits the mevalonate pathway causing reduction of non-sterol isoprenoid levels and protein prenylation [106]. The dysregulation of the mevalonate pathway in AD may affect neurons and glia in different ways. Our findings suggest that inhibition of the mevalonate pathway will take place specifically in cells that accumulate Aβ, most likely neurons. Depending on the size of the cell population that contains intracellular Aβ, this might or might not impact the overall content of cholesterol and isoprenoids in the brain. The decreased synthesis of cholesterol in neurons may be compensated by synthesis in astrocytes [21]. In addition, an interesting model has been proposed in which SREBPs in astrocytes would be involved in synthesis of fatty acids and perhaps other lipids for neuronal supply [424]. According to this model, glia SREBPs may work as control points of neuronal function, providing neurons with appropriate lipids when neurons cannot make their own. The shuttle of non-sterol isoprenoids and 25-EC from astrocytes to neurons has been suggested [206, 351]. These possible homeostatic mechanisms should be taken in consideration when brain levels of lipids are analyzed. The increase of non-sterol isoprenoids in AD brains, if confirmed in a larger cohort, may represent an astrocytic attempt to compensate for the decrease in SREBP-dependent metabolic pathways in neurons. Compensatory attempt mechanisms in brain cholesterol homeostasis in AD have been described before. The amount of CYP46, the enzyme that converts cholesterol into 24-HC decreases in neuronal cells in AD brains, but this decrease is at least in part compensated for by an induction of the enzyme in glial cells [425]. In conclusion, our knowledge on the impairment of the mevalonate pathway in AD is still very limited. The extremely complex regulation of this pathway represents a challenge for the complete understanding of the defects present during AD. Defects at the cellular level are important but ultimately we need to comprehend how the interaction neuron-glia regulates the mevalonate pathway in the brain.

5. Abreviations

24-HC: 24(S)-hydroxycholesterol; **25-HC**: 24(S),25-epoxycholesterol; **7-DHC**: 7-dehydrocholesterol; **ABC**: adenosine triphosphate-binding cassette transporter; **ACAT**: acyl coA-cholesterol acyltransferase; **AD**: Alzheimer's disease; **AMPK**: adenosine monophosphate-activated protein kinase; **apoE4**: apolipoprotein E ε4; **Aβ**: amyloid-beta peptide; **BACE-1**: beta-site APP cleaving enzyme 1; **BBB**: blood-brain-barrier; **CNS**: central nervous system; **CoA**: coenzyme A; **CSF**: cerebrospinal fluid; **CYP46A1**: 24-hydroxylase; **DHCR24**: 24-dehydrocholesterol reductase; **DMPP**: dimethylallyl pyrophosphate; **DOS**: dioxidosqualene; **FOH**: farnesol; **FPP**: farnesyl pyrophosphate; **FPPS**: FPP synthase; **FTase**: farnesyl protein transferase; **GDP**: guanosine diphosphate; **GGOH**: geranylgeraniol; **GGPP**: geranylgeranyl pyrophosphate; **GGPPS**: GGPP synthase; **GGTase-I**: geranylgeranyl transferase type I; **GPP**: geranyl pyrophosphate; **HMG**: 3-hydroxy-3-methylglutaryl-CoA; **IDE**: insulin degrading enzyme; **Insig**: insulin-induced gene; **IPP**: isopentenylpyrophosphate; **LTP**: long-term potentiation; **LXR**: liver-X-receptor; **MCI**: mild cognitive impairment; **MK**: mevalonate kinase; **MOS**: monooxidosqualene; **NFT**: neurofibrillary tangle; **NPC**: Niemann-Pick type C; **REST**: RE1-silencing transcription factor; **SCAP**: SREBP-cleavage activating protein; **SREBP**: sterol-regulatory element binding protein; **TRP**: transient receptor potential

Author details

Amany Mohamed[1,2], Kevan Smith[1,2] and Elena Posse de Chaves[1,2*]

*Address all correspondence to: elena.chaves@ualberta.ca

1 Department of Pharmacology, University of Alberta, Edmonton, AB, Canada

2 Neuroscience and Mental Health Institute, University of Alberta, Edmonton, AB, Canada

References

[1] O'Brien, J.S. and E.L. Sampson, *Lipid composition of the normal human brain: gray matter, white matter, and myelin.* J Lipid Res, 1965. 6(4): p. 537-44.

[2] Dietschy, J.M. and S.D. Turley, *Thematic review series: brain Lipids. Cholesterol metabolism in the central nervous system during early development and in the mature animal.* J Lipid Res, 2004. 45(8): p. 1375-97.

[3] Dietschy, J.M., *Central nervous system: cholesterol turnover, brain development and neurodegeneration.* Biol Chem, 2009. 390(4): p. 287-93.

[4] Corder, E.H., et al., *Gene dose of apolipoprotein E type 4 allele and the risk of Alzheimer's disease in late onset families.* Science, 1993. 261(5123): p. 921-3.

[5] Martins, I.J., et al., *Cholesterol metabolism and transport in the pathogenesis of Alzheimer's disease.* J Neurochem, 2009. 111(6): p. 1275-308.

[6] Carter, C.J., *Convergence of genes implicated in Alzheimer's disease on the cerebral cholesterol shuttle: APP, cholesterol, lipoproteins, and atherosclerosis.* Neurochemistry international, 2007. 50(1): p. 12-38.

[7] Wollmer, M.A., *Cholesterol-related genes in Alzheimer's disease.* Biochim Biophys Acta, 2010. 1801(8): p. 762-73.

[8] Wollmer, M.A., et al., *Association study of cholesterol-related genes in Alzheimer's disease.* Neurogenetics, 2007. 8(3): p. 179-88.

[9] Bertram, L., C.M. Lill, and R.E. Tanzi, *The genetics of Alzheimer disease: back to the future.* Neuron, 2010. 68(2): p. 270-81.

[10] Di Paolo, G. and T.W. Kim, *Linking lipids to Alzheimer's disease: cholesterol and beyond.* Nat Rev Neurosci, 2011. 12(5): p. 284-96.

[11] Posse de Chaves, E., *Reciprocal regulation of cholesterol and beta amyloid at the subcellular level in Alzheimer's disease.* Can J Physiol Pharmacol, 2012. 90(6): p. 753-64.

[12] Maulik, M., et al., *Role of cholesterol in APP metabolism and its significance in Alzheimer's disease pathogenesis.* Mol Neurobiol, 2013. 47(1): p. 37-63.

[13] Jick, H., et al., *Statins and the risk of dementia.* Lancet, 2000. 356(9242): p. 1627-31.

[14] Wolozin, B., et al., *Decreased prevalence of Alzheimer disease associated with 3-hydroxy-3-methyglutaryl coenzyme A reductase inhibitors.* Arch Neurol, 2000. 57(10): p. 1439-43.

[15] Arvanitakis, Z. and D.S. Knopman, *Clinical trial efforts in Alzheimer disease: why test statins?* Neurology, 2010. 74(12): p. 945-6.

[16] Rea, T.D., et al., *Statin use and the risk of incident dementia: the Cardiovascular Health Study.* Arch Neurol, 2005. 62(7): p. 1047-51.

[17] Kandiah, N. and H.H. Feldman, *Therapeutic potential of statins in Alzheimer's disease.* J Neurol Sci, 2009. 283(1-2): p. 230-4.

[18] Shepardson, N.E., G.M. Shankar, and D.J. Selkoe, *Cholesterol level and statin use in Alzheimer disease: I. Review of epidemiological and preclinical studies.* Archives of neurology, 2011. 68(10): p. 1239-44.

[19] Shepardson, N.E., G.M. Shankar, and D.J. Selkoe, *Cholesterol level and statin use in Alzheimer disease: II. Review of human trials and recommendations.* Arch Neurol, 2011. 68(11): p. 1385-92.

[20] Jones, L., et al., *Genetic evidence implicates the immune system and cholesterol metabolism in the aetiology of Alzheimer's disease.* PloS one, 2010. 5(11): p. e13950.

[21] Pfrieger, F.W. and N. Ungerer, *Cholesterol metabolism in neurons and astrocytes.* Progress in lipid research, 2011. 50(4): p. 357-371.

[22] Thelen, K.M., et al., *Cholesterol synthesis rate in human hippocampus declines with aging.* Neurosci Lett, 2006. 403(1-2): p. 15-9.

[23] Waterham, H.R., *Defects of cholesterol biosynthesis.* FEBS letters, 2006. 580(23): p. 5442-9.

[24] Bjorkhem, I., V. Leoni, and S. Meaney, *Genetic connections between neurological disorders and cholesterol metabolism.* Journal of lipid research, 2010. 51(9): p. 2489-503.

[25] Nieweg, K., H. Schaller, and F.W. Pfrieger, *Marked differences in cholesterol synthesis between neurons and glial cells from postnatal rats.* J Neurochem, 2009. 109(1): p. 125-34.

[26] Ullian, E.M., K.S. Christopherson, and B.A. Barres, *Role for glia in synaptogenesis.* Glia, 2004. 47(3): p. 209-16.

[27] Mauch, D.H., et al., *CNS synaptogenesis promoted by glia-derived cholesterol.* Science, 2001. 294(5545): p. 1354-7.

[28] Funfschilling, U., et al., *Survival of adult neurons lacking cholesterol synthesis in vivo.* BMC Neurosci, 2007. 8: p. 1.

[29] Valdez, C.M., et al., *Cholesterol homeostasis markers are localized to mouse hippocampal pyramidal and granule layers.* Hippocampus, 2010.

[30] Wahrle, S.E., et al., *ABCA1 is required for normal central nervous system ApoE levels and for lipidation of astrocyte-secreted apoE.* The Journal of Biological Chemistry, 2004. 279(39): p. 40987-93.

[31] Holtzman, D.M., J. Herz, and G. Bu, *Apolipoprotein E and apolipoprotein E receptors: normal biology and roles in Alzheimer disease.* Cold Spring Harb Perspect Med, 2012. 2(3): p. a006312.

[32] Pitas, R.E., et al., *Lipoproteins and their receptors in the central nervous system. Characterization of the lipoproteins in cerebrospinal fluid and identification of apolipoprotein B,E(LDL) receptors in the brain.* J Biol Chem, 1987. 262(29): p. 14352-60.

[33] LaDu, M.J., et al., *Nascent astrocyte particles differ from lipoproteins in CSF.* J Neurochem, 1998. 70(5): p. 2070-81.

[34] Bjorkhem, I. and S. Meaney, *Brain cholesterol: long secret life behind a barrier.* Arterioscler Thromb Vasc Biol, 2004. 24(5): p. 806-15.

[35] Lutjohann, D., et al., *Cholesterol homeostasis in human brain: evidence for an age-dependent flux of 24S-hydroxycholesterol from the brain into the circulation.* Proc Natl Acad Sci U S A, 1996. 93(18): p. 9799-804.

[36] Lund, E.G., J.M. Guileyardo, and D.W. Russell, *cDNA cloning of cholesterol 24-hydroxylase, a mediator of cholesterol homeostasis in the brain.* Proc Natl Acad Sci U S A, 1999. 96(13): p. 7238-43.

[37] Ramirez, D.M., S. Andersson, and D.W. Russell, *Neuronal expression and subcellular localization of cholesterol 24-hydroxylase in the mouse brain.* J Comp Neurol, 2008. 507(5): p. 1676-93.

[38] Abildayeva, K., et al., *24(S)-hydroxycholesterol participates in a liver X receptor-controlled pathway in astrocytes that regulates apolipoprotein E-mediated cholesterol efflux.* J Biol Chem, 2006. 281(18): p. 12799-808.

[39] Buhman, K.F., M. Accad, and R.V. Farese, *Mammalian acyl-CoA:cholesterol acyltransferases.* Biochim Biophys Acta, 2000. 1529(1-3): p. 142-54.

[40] Johnson, R.C. and S.N. Shah, *Cholesterol ester metabolizing enzymes in human brain: properties, subcellular distribution and relative levels in various diseased conditions.* J Neurochem, 1978. 31(4): p. 895-902.

[41] Bryleva, E.Y., et al., *ACAT1 gene ablation increases 24(S)-hydroxycholesterol content in the brain and ameliorates amyloid pathology in mice with AD.* Proc Natl Acad Sci U S A, 2010. 107(7): p. 3081-6.

[42] Huttunen, H.J. and D.M. Kovacs, *ACAT as a drug target for Alzheimer's disease.* Neurodegener Dis, 2008. 5(3-4): p. 212-4.

[43] Rubinsztein, D.C. and D.F. Easton, *Apolipoprotein E genetic variation and Alzheimer's disease. a meta-analysis.* Dement Geriatr Cogn Disord, 1999. 10(3): p. 199-209.

[44] Harold, D., et al., *Genome-wide association study identifies variants at CLU and PICALM associated with Alzheimer's disease.* Nat Genet, 2009. 41(10): p. 1088-93.

[45] Katzov, H., et al., *Genetic variants of ABCA1 modify Alzheimer disease risk and quantitative traits related to beta-amyloid metabolism.* Hum Mutat, 2004. 23(4): p. 358-67.

[46]   Sundar, P.D., et al., *Gender-specific association of ATP-binding cassette transporter I (ABCA1) polymorphisms with the risk of late-onset Alzheimer's disease.* Neurobiology of Aging, 2007. 28(6): p. 856-862.

[47]   Li, Y.H., et al., *Association of ABCA1 with late-onset Alzheimer's disease is not observed in a case-control study.* Neuroscience Letters, 2004. 366(3): p. 268-271.

[48]   Wollmer, M.A., et al., *ABCA1 modulates CSF cholesterol levels and influences the age at onset of Alzheimer's disease.* Neurobiology of aging, 2003. 24(3): p. 421-6.

[49]   Kolsch, H., et al., *Polymorphism in the cholesterol 24S-hydroxylase gene is associated with Alzheimer's disease.* Molecular Psychiatry, 2002. 7(8): p. 899-902.

[50]   Desai, P., S.T. DeKosky, and M.I. Kamboh, *Genetic variation in the cholesterol 24-hydroxylase (CYP46) gene and the risk of Alzheimer's disease.* Neuroscience letters, 2002. 328(1): p. 9-12.

[51]   Papassotiropoulos, A., et al., *Increased brain beta-amyloid load, phosphorylated tau, and risk of Alzheimer disease associated with an intronic CYP46 polymorphism.* Arch Neurol, 2003. 60(1): p. 29-35.

[52]   Johansson, A., et al., *Variants of CYP46A1 may interact with age and APOE to influence CSF A beta 42 levels in Alzheimer's disease.* Human Genetics, 2004. 114(6): p. 581-587.

[53]   Kolsch, H., et al., *Association of the C766T polymorphism of the low-density lipoprotein receptor-related protein gene with Alzheimer's disease.* Am J Med Genet B Neuropsychiatr Genet, 2003. 121B(1): p. 128-30.

[54]   Causevic, M., et al., *Lack of association between the levels of the low-density lipoprotein receptor-related protein (LRP) and either Alzheimer dementia or LRP exon 3 genotype.* Journal of Neuropathology and Experimental Neurology, 2003. 62(10): p. 999-1005.

[55]   Lendon, C.L., et al., *Genetic association studies between dementia of the Alzheimer's type and three receptors for apolipoprotein E in a Caucasian population.* Neuroscience Letters, 1997. 222(3): p. 187-190.

[56]   Wollmer, M.A., et al., *Genetic association of acyl-coenzyme A: cholesterol acyltransferase with cerebrospinal fluid cholesterol levels, brain amyloid load, and risk for Alzheimer's disease.* Molecular psychiatry, 2003. 8(6): p. 635-8.

[57]   Bloch, K., *The biological synthesis of cholesterol.* Science, 1965. 150(3692): p. 19-28.

[58]   Panda, T., et al., *Kinetic Mechanisms of Cholesterol Synthesis: A Review.* Industrial & Engineering Chemistry Research, 2011. 50(23): p. 12847-12864.

[59]   Miziorko, H.M., *Enzymes of the mevalonate pathway of isoprenoid biosynthesis.* Arch Biochem Biophys, 2011. 505(2): p. 131-43.

[60]   Korade, Z., et al., *Expression and p75 neurotrophin receptor dependence of cholesterol synthetic enzymes in adult mouse brain.* Neurobiology of aging, 2007. 28(10): p. 1522-31.

[61] Levin, M.S., et al., *Developmental changes in the expression of genes involved in cholesterol biosynthesis and lipid transport in human and rat fetal and neonatal livers.* Biochim Biophys Acta, 1989. 1003(3): p. 293-300.

[62] Ness, G.C., *Developmental regulation of the expression of genes encoding proteins involved in cholesterol homeostasis.* Am J Med Genet, 1994. 50(4): p. 355-7.

[63] Kanungo, S., et al., *Sterol metabolism disorders and neurodevelopment-an update.* Dev Disabil Res Rev, 2013. 17(3): p. 197-210.

[64] Cedazo-Minguez, A., M.A. Ismail, and L. Mateos, *Plasma cholesterol and risk for late-onset Alzheimer's disease.* Expert review of neurotherapeutics, 2011. 11(4): p. 495-8.

[65] Rockwood, K., *Epidemiological and clinical trials evidence about a preventive role for statins in Alzheimer's disease.* Acta Neurol Scand Suppl, 2006. 185: p. 71-7.

[66] Horton, J.D., J.L. Goldstein, and M.S. Brown, *SREBPs: activators of the complete program of cholesterol and fatty acid synthesis in the liver.* The Journal of clinical investigation, 2002. 109(9): p. 1125-31.

[67] Horton, J.D., et al., *Combined analysis of oligonucleotide microarray data from transgenic and knockout mice identifies direct SREBP target genes.* Proceedings of the National Academy of Sciences of the United States of America, 2003. 100(21): p. 12027-32.

[68] Brown, M.S. and J.L. Goldstein, *The SREBP pathway: regulation of cholesterol metabolism by proteolysis of a membrane-bound transcription factor.* Cell, 1997. 89(3): p. 331-40.

[69] Rawson, R.B., *Control of lipid metabolism by regulated intramembrane proteolysis of sterol regulatory element binding proteins (SREBPs).* Biochem Soc Symp, 2003(70): p. 221-31.

[70] Horton, A.C. and M.D. Ehlers, *Dual modes of endoplasmic reticulum-to-Golgi transport in dendrites revealed by live-cell imaging.* J Neurosci, 2003. 23(15): p. 6188-99.

[71] Suzuki, R., et al., *Reduction of the cholesterol sensor SCAP in the brains of mice causes impaired synaptic transmission and altered cognitive function.* PLoS Biol, 2013. 11(4): p. e1001532.

[72] Espenshade, P.J., et al., *Autocatalytic processing of site-1 protease removes propeptide and permits cleavage of sterol regulatory element-binding proteins.* J Biol Chem, 1999. 274(32): p. 22795-804.

[73] Zelenski, N.G., et al., *Membrane topology of S2P, a protein required for intramembranous cleavage of sterol regulatory element-binding proteins.* J Biol Chem, 1999. 274(31): p. 21973-80.

[74] McPherson, R. and A. Gauthier, *Molecular regulation of SREBP function: the Insig-SCAP connection and isoform-specific modulation of lipid synthesis.* Biochem Cell Biol, 2004. 82(1): p. 201-11.

[75] Inoue, J., R. Sato, and M. Maeda, *Multiple DNA elements for sterol regulatory element-binding protein and NF-Y are responsible for sterol-regulated transcription of the genes for*

human 3-hydroxy-3-methylglutaryl coenzyme A synthase and squalene synthase. J Biochem, 1998. 123(6): p. 1191-8.

[76] Yieh, L., H.B. Sanchez, and T.F. Osborne, *Domains of transcription factor Sp1 required for synergistic activation with sterol regulatory element binding protein 1 of low density lipo-protein receptor promoter.* Proc Natl Acad Sci U S A, 1995. 92(13): p. 6102-6.

[77] Zerenturk, E.J., L.J. Sharpe, and A.J. Brown, *Sterols regulate 3beta-hydroxysterol Del-ta24-reductase (DHCR24) via dual sterol regulatory elements: cooperative induction of key enzymes in lipid synthesis by Sterol Regulatory Element Binding Proteins.* Biochim Bio-phys Acta, 2012. 1821(10): p. 1350-60.

[78] Horie, T., et al., *MicroRNA-33 encoded by an intron of sterol regulatory element-binding protein 2 (Srebp2) regulates HDL in vivo.* Proceedings of the National Academy of Sci-ences of the United States of America, 2010. 107(40): p. 17321-6.

[79] Gerin, I., et al., *Expression of miR-33 from an SREBP2 intron inhibits cholesterol export and fatty acid oxidation.* The Journal of Biological Chemistry, 2010. 285(44): p. 33652-61.

[80] Najafi-Shoushtari, S.H., et al., *MicroRNA-33 and the SREBP host genes cooperate to con-trol cholesterol homeostasis.* Science, 2010. 328(5985): p. 1566-9.

[81] Marquart, T.J., et al., *miR-33 links SREBP-2 induction to repression of sterol transporters.* Proceedings of the National Academy of Sciences of the United States of America, 2010. 107(27): p. 12228-32.

[82] Rayner, K.J., et al., *MiR-33 contributes to the regulation of cholesterol homeostasis.* Science, 2010. 328(5985): p. 1570-3.

[83] Bommer, G.T. and O.A. MacDougald, *Regulation of lipid homeostasis by the bifunctional SREBF2-miR33a locus.* Cell metabolism, 2011. 13(3): p. 241-7.

[84] Adlakha, Y.K., et al., *Pro-apoptotic miRNA-128-2 modulates ABCA1, ABCG1 and RXRal-pha expression and cholesterol homeostasis.* Cell Death Dis, 2013. 4: p. e780.

[85] Kim, J.H. and W.Y. Ong, *Localization of the transcription factor, sterol regulatory element binding protein-2 (SREBP-2) in the normal rat brain and changes after kainate-induced exci-totoxic injury.* J Chem Neuroanat, 2009. 37(2): p. 71-7.

[86] Radhakrishnan, A., et al., *Switch-like control of SREBP-2 transport triggered by small changes in ER cholesterol: a delicate balance.* Cell Metab, 2008. 8(6): p. 512-21.

[87] Brown, A.J., et al., *Cholesterol addition to ER membranes alters conformation of SCAP, the SREBP escort protein that regulates cholesterol metabolism.* Mol Cell, 2002. 10(2): p. 237-45.

[88] Radhakrishnan, A., et al., *Direct binding of cholesterol to the purified membrane region of SCAP: mechanism for a sterol-sensing domain.* Mol Cell, 2004. 15(2): p. 259-68.

[89] Yang, T., et al., *Crucial step in cholesterol homeostasis: sterols promote binding of SCAP to INSIG-1, a membrane protein that facilitates retention of SREBPs in ER.* Cell, 2002. 110(4): p. 489-500.

[90] Rodriguez-Acebes, S., et al., *Desmosterol can replace cholesterol in sustaining cell proliferation and regulating the SREBP pathway in a sterol-Delta24-reductase-deficient cell line.* Biochem J, 2009. 420(2): p. 305-15.

[91] Song, B.L., N.B. Javitt, and R.A. DeBose-Boyd, *Insig-mediated degradation of HMG CoA reductase stimulated by lanosterol, an intermediate in the synthesis of cholesterol.* Cell Metab, 2005. 1(3): p. 179-89.

[92] Radhakrishnan, A., et al., *Sterol-regulated transport of SREBPs from endoplasmic reticulum to Golgi: oxysterols block transport by binding to Insig.* Proc Natl Acad Sci U S A, 2007. 104(16): p. 6511-8.

[93] Sato, R., et al., *Sterol-dependent transcriptional regulation of sterol regulatory element-binding protein-2.* J Biol Chem, 1996. 271(43): p. 26461-4.

[94] Jeon, T.I., et al., *An SREBP-responsive microRNA operon contributes to a regulatory loop for intracellular lipid homeostasis.* Cell Metab, 2013. 18(1): p. 51-61.

[95] Hu, Y.W., L. Zheng, and Q. Wang, *Regulation of cholesterol homeostasis by liver X receptors.* Clin Chim Acta, 2010. 411(9-10): p. 617-25.

[96] Beaven, S.W. and P. Tontonoz, *Nuclear receptors in lipid metabolism: targeting the heart of dyslipidemia.* Annual review of medicine, 2006. 57: p. 313-29.

[97] Jakobsson, T., et al., *Liver X receptor biology and pharmacology: new pathways, challenges and opportunities.* Trends Pharmacol Sci, 2012. 33(7): p. 394-404.

[98] Whitney, K.D., et al., *Regulation of cholesterol homeostasis by the liver X receptors in the central nervous system.* Mol Endocrinol, 2002. 16(6): p. 1378-85.

[99] Wong, J., C.M. Quinn, and A.J. Brown, *SREBP-2 positively regulates transcription of the cholesterol efflux gene, ABCA1, by generating oxysterol ligands for LXR.* Biochem J, 2006. 400(3): p. 485-91.

[100] Eckert, G.P., et al., *Regulation of central nervous system cholesterol homeostasis by the liver X receptor agonist TO-901317.* Neurosci Lett, 2007. 423(1): p. 47-52.

[101] Zelcer, N., et al., *LXR regulates cholesterol uptake through Idol-dependent ubiquitination of the LDL receptor.* Science, 2009. 325(5936): p. 100-4.

[102] Wang, Y., et al., *Regulation of cholesterologenesis by the oxysterol receptor, LXRalpha.* J Biol Chem, 2008. 283(39): p. 26332-9.

[103] Wang, L., et al., *Liver X receptors in the central nervous system: from lipid homeostasis to neuronal degeneration.* Proc Natl Acad Sci U S A, 2002. 99(21): p. 13878-83.

[104] Xiong, H., et al., *Cholesterol retention in Alzheimer's brain is responsible for high beta- and gamma-secretase activities and Abeta production.* Neurobiol Dis, 2008. 29(3): p. 422-37.

[105] Blalock, E.M., et al., *Incipient Alzheimer's disease: microarray correlation analyses reveal major transcriptional and tumor suppressor responses.* Proc Natl Acad Sci U S A, 2004. 101(7): p. 2173-8.

[106] Mohamed, A., et al., *beta-amyloid inhibits protein prenylation and induces cholesterol sequestration by impairing SREBP-2 cleavage.* J Neurosci, 2012. 32(19): p. 6490-500.

[107] Mohamed, A.a.P.d.C., EI, *Abeta Inhibits SREBP-2 Cleavage by Reducing Cellular Levels of Activated Akt* The 11th International Conference on Alzheimer's and Parkinson's Diseases, 2013- Florence, Italy, March 6-10.

[108] Pierrot, N., et al., *Amyloid precursor protein controls cholesterol turnover needed for neuronal activity.* EMBO Mol Med, 2013. 5(4): p. 608-25.

[109] Ferguson, J.J., I.F. Durr, and H. Rudney, *The Biosynthesis of Mevalonic Acid.* Proc Natl Acad Sci U S A, 1959. 45(4): p. 499-504.

[110] Rodwell, V.W., J.L. Nordstrom, and J.J. Mitschelen, *Regulation of HMG-CoA reductase.* Adv Lipid Res, 1976. 14: p. 1-74.

[111] Goldstein, J.L. and M.S. Brown, *Regulation of the mevalonate pathway.* Nature, 1990. 343(6257): p. 425-30.

[112] Simmons, C.R., et al., *Evaluation of the global association between cholesterol-associated polymorphisms and Alzheimer's disease suggests a role for rs3846662 and HMGCR splicing in disease risk.* Molecular neurodegeneration, 2011. 6: p. 62.

[113] Kovacs, W.J., et al., *Purification of brain peroxisomes and localization of 3-hydroxy-3-methylglutaryl coenzyme A reductase.* Eur J Biochem, 2001. 268(18): p. 4850-9.

[114] Horvat, S., J. McWhir, and D. Rozman, *Defects in cholesterol synthesis genes in mouse and in humans: lessons for drug development and safer treatments.* Drug Metab Rev, 2011. 43(1): p. 69-90.

[115] Tchen, T.T., *Mevalonic kinase: purification and properties.* J Biol Chem, 1958. 233(5): p. 1100-3.

[116] van der Burgh, R., et al., *Mevalonate kinase deficiency, a metabolic autoinflammatory disease.* Clin Immunol, 2013. 147(3): p. 197-206.

[117] Tada, M. and F. Lynen, *[On the biosynthesis of terpenes. XIV. On the determination of phosphomevalonic acid kinase and pyrophosphomevalonic acid decarboxylase in cell extracts].* J Biochem, 1961. 49: p. 758-64.

[118] Agranoff, B.W., et al., *Biosynthesis of terpenes. VII. Isopentenyl pyrophosphate isomerase.* J Biol Chem, 1960. 235: p. 326-32.

[119] Moosmann, B. and C. Behl, *Selenoproteins, cholesterol-lowering drugs, and the consequences: revisiting of the mevalonate pathway.* Trends Cardiovasc Med, 2004. 14(7): p. 273-81.

[120] Warner, G.J., et al., *Inhibition of selenoprotein synthesis by selenocysteine tRNA[Ser]Sec lacking isopentenyladenosine.* J Biol Chem, 2000. 275(36): p. 28110-9.

[121] Bellinger, F.P., et al., *Regulation and function of selenoproteins in human disease.* Biochem J, 2009. 422(1): p. 11-22.

[122] Zhang, S., C. Rocourt, and W.H. Cheng, *Selenoproteins and the aging brain.* Mech Ageing Dev, 2010. 131(4): p. 253-60.

[123] Wirth, E.K., et al., *Neuronal selenoprotein expression is required for interneuron development and prevents seizures and neurodegeneration.* FASEB J, 2010. 24(3): p. 844-52.

[124] Seeher, S., et al., *Impaired selenoprotein expression in brain triggers striatal neuronal loss leading to co-ordination defects in mice.* Biochem J, 2014. 462(1): p. 67-75.

[125] Moosmann, B. and C. Behl, *Selenoprotein synthesis and side-effects of statins.* Lancet, 2004. 363(9412): p. 892-4.

[126] Bang, S., et al., *Isopentenyl pyrophosphate is a novel antinociceptive substance that inhibits TRPV3 and TRPA1 ion channels.* Pain, 2011. 152(5): p. 1156-64.

[127] Bang, S., et al., *Nociceptive and pro-inflammatory effects of dimethylallyl pyrophosphate via TRPV4 activation.* Br J Pharmacol, 2012. 166(4): p. 1433-43.

[128] Holstein, S.A. and R.J. Hohl, *Isoprenoids: remarkable diversity of form and function.* Lipids, 2004. 39(4): p. 293-309.

[129] Hooff, G.P., et al., *Isoprenoids, small GTPases and Alzheimer's disease.* Biochim Biophys Acta, 2010. 1801(8): p. 896-905.

[130] Wang, K.C. and S. Ohnuma, *Isoprenyl diphosphate synthases.* Biochim Biophys Acta, 2000. 1529(1-3): p. 33-48.

[131] Vallett, S.M., et al., *A direct role for sterol regulatory element binding protein in activation of 3-hydroxy-3-methylglutaryl coenzyme A reductase gene.* J Biol Chem, 1996. 271(21): p. 12247-53.

[132] Sharpe, L.J. and A.J. Brown, *Controlling Cholesterol Synthesis beyond 3-Hydroxy-3-methylglutaryl-CoA Reductase (HMGCR).* J Biol Chem, 2013. 288(26): p. 18707-15.

[133] Medina, M.W., et al., *Coordinately regulated alternative splicing of genes involved in cholesterol biosynthesis and uptake.* PLoS One, 2011. 6(4): p. e19420.

[134] Nakanishi, M., J.L. Goldstein, and M.S. Brown, *Multivalent control of 3-hydroxy-3-methylglutaryl coenzyme A reductase. Mevalonate-derived product inhibits translation of mRNA and accelerates degradation of enzyme.* J Biol Chem, 1988. 263(18): p. 8929-37.

[135] Peffley, D. and M. Sinensky, *Regulation of 3-hydroxy-3-methylglutaryl coenzyme A reductase synthesis by a non-sterol mevalonate-derived product in Mev-1 cells. Apparent translational control.* J Biol Chem, 1985. 260(18): p. 9949-52.

[136] Straka, M.S. and S.R. Panini, *Post-transcriptional regulation of 3-hydroxy-3-methylglutaryl coenzyme A reductase by mevalonate.* Arch Biochem Biophys, 1995. 317(1): p. 235-43.

[137] Peffley, D.M. and A.K. Gayen, *Plant-derived monoterpenes suppress hamster kidney cell 3-hydroxy-3-methylglutaryl coenzyme a reductase synthesis at the post-transcriptional level.* J Nutr, 2003. 133(1): p. 38-44.

[138] Peffley, D.M. and A.K. Gayen, *Mevalonate regulates polysome distribution and blocks translation-dependent suppression of 3-hydroxy-3-methylglutaryl coenzyme A reductase mRNA: relationship to translational control.* Somat Cell Mol Genet, 1995. 21(3): p. 189-204.

[139] Ching, Y.P., S.P. Davies, and D.G. Hardie, *Analysis of the specificity of the AMP-activated protein kinase by site-directed mutagenesis of bacterially expressed 3-hydroxy 3-methylglutaryl-CoA reductase, using a single primer variant of the unique-site-elimination method.* Eur J Biochem, 1996. 237(3): p. 800-8.

[140] Clarke, P.R. and D.G. Hardie, *Regulation of HMG-CoA reductase: identification of the site phosphorylated by the AMP-activated protein kinase in vitro and in intact rat liver.* EMBO J, 1990. 9(8): p. 2439-46.

[141] Gaussin, V., et al., *Distinct type-2A protein phosphatases activate HMGCoA reductase and acetyl-CoA carboxylase in liver.* FEBS Lett, 1997. 413(1): p. 115-8.

[142] Cook, M., et al., *Increased RhoA prenylation in the loechrig (loe) mutant leads to progressive neurodegeneration.* PLoS One, 2012. 7(9): p. e44440.

[143] Lu, J., et al., *Quercetin activates AMP-activated protein kinase by reducing PP2C expression protecting old mouse brain against high cholesterol-induced neurotoxicity.* The Journal of pathology, 2010. 222(2): p. 199-212.

[144] Song, B.L., N. Sever, and R.A. DeBose-Boyd, *Gp78, a membrane-anchored ubiquitin ligase, associates with Insig-1 and couples sterol-regulated ubiquitination to degradation of HMG CoA reductase.* Mol Cell, 2005. 19(6): p. 829-40.

[145] Jo, Y., et al., *Sterol-induced degradation of HMG CoA reductase depends on interplay of two Insigs and two ubiquitin ligases, gp78 and Trc8.* Proc Natl Acad Sci U S A, 2011. 108(51): p. 20503-8.

[146] Zelcer, N., et al., *The E3 ubiquitin ligase MARCH6 degrades squalene monooxygenase and affects 3-hydroxy-3-methyl-glutaryl coenzyme A reductase and the cholesterol synthesis pathway.* Mol Cell Biol, 2014. 34(7): p. 1262-70.

[147] Sever, N., et al., *Insig-dependent ubiquitination and degradation of mammalian 3-hydroxy-3-methylglutaryl-CoA reductase stimulated by sterols and geranylgeraniol.* The Journal of Biological Chemistry, 2003. 278(52): p. 52479-90.

[148] Hua, X., et al., *Sterol resistance in CHO cells traced to point mutation in SREBP cleavage-activating protein.* Cell, 1996. 87(3): p. 415-26.

[149] Sever, N., et al., *Accelerated degradation of HMG CoA reductase mediated by binding of insig-1 to its sterol-sensing domain.* Molecular cell, 2003. 11(1): p. 25-33.

[150] Song, B.L. and R.A. DeBose-Boyd, *Ubiquitination of 3-hydroxy-3-methylglutaryl-CoA reductase in permeabilized cells mediated by cytosolic E1 and a putative membrane-bound ubiquitin ligase.* J Biol Chem, 2004. 279(27): p. 28798-806.

[151] DeBose-Boyd, R.A., *Feedback regulation of cholesterol synthesis: sterol-accelerated ubiquitination and degradation of HMG CoA reductase.* Cell research, 2008. 18(6): p. 609-21.

[152] Lange, Y., et al., *Effectors of rapid homeostatic responses of endoplasmic reticulum cholesterol and 3-hydroxy-3-methylglutaryl-CoA reductase.* J Biol Chem, 2008. 283(3): p. 1445-55.

[153] Forman, B.M., et al., *The orphan nuclear receptor LXRalpha is positively and negatively regulated by distinct products of mevalonate metabolism.* Proc Natl Acad Sci U S A, 1997. 94(20): p. 10588-93.

[154] Gan, X., et al., *Dual mechanisms of ABCA1 regulation by geranylgeranyl pyrophosphate.* J Biol Chem, 2001. 276(52): p. 48702-8.

[155] Leichner, G.S., et al., *Metabolically Regulated Endoplasmic Reticulum-associated Degradation of 3-Hydroxy-3-methylglutaryl-CoA Reductase: EVIDENCE FOR REQUIREMENT OF A GERANYLGERANYLATED PROTEIN.* The Journal of Biological Chemistry, 2011. 286(37): p. 32150-61.

[156] Meigs, T.E., D.S. Roseman, and R.D. Simoni, *Regulation of 3-hydroxy-3-methylglutaryl-coenzyme A reductase degradation by the nonsterol mevalonate metabolite farnesol in vivo.* J Biol Chem, 1996. 271(14): p. 7916-22.

[157] Meigs, T.E. and R.D. Simoni, *Farnesol as a regulator of HMG-CoA reductase degradation: characterization and role of farnesyl pyrophosphatase.* Arch Biochem Biophys, 1997. 345(1): p. 1-9.

[158] Correll, C.C., L. Ng, and P.A. Edwards, *Identification of farnesol as the non-sterol derivative of mevalonic acid required for the accelerated degradation of 3-hydroxy-3-methylglutaryl-coenzyme A reductase.* J Biol Chem, 1994. 269(26): p. 17390-3.

[159] Dorsey, J.K. and J.W. Porter, *The inhibition of mevalonic kinase by geranyl and farnesyl pyrophosphates.* J Biol Chem, 1968. 243(18): p. 4667-70.

[160] Hinson, D.D., et al., *Post-translational regulation of mevalonate kinase by intermediates of the cholesterol and nonsterol isoprene biosynthetic pathways.* J Lipid Res, 1997. 38(11): p. 2216-23.

[161] Vanmierlo, T., et al., *Alterations in brain cholesterol metabolism in the APPSLxPS1mut mouse, a model for Alzheimer's disease.* J Alzheimers Dis, 2010. 19(1): p. 117-27.

[162] Licastro, F., et al., *Genetic risk profiles for Alzheimer's disease: integration of APOE genotype and variants that up-regulate inflammation.* Neurobiol Aging, 2007. 28(11): p. 1637-43.

[163] Porcellini, E., et al., *The hydroxy-methyl-glutaryl CoA reductase promoter polymorphism is associated with Alzheimer's risk and cognitive deterioration.* Neuroscience Letters, 2007. 416(1): p. 66-70.

[164] Rodriguez-Rodriguez, E., et al., *Interaction between HMGCR and ABCA1 cholesterol-related genes modulates Alzheimer's disease risk.* Brain Res, 2009. 1280: p. 166-71.

[165] Keller, L., et al., *A functional polymorphism in the HMGCR promoter affects transcriptional activity but not the risk for Alzheimer disease in Swedish populations.* Brain Res, 2010. 1344: p. 185-91.

[166] Leduc, V., et al., *HMGCR is a genetic modifier for risk, age of onset and MCI conversion to Alzheimer's disease in a three cohorts study.* Mol Psychiatry, 2014.

[167] Trapani, L. and V. Pallottini, *Age-Related Hypercholesterolemia and HMG-CoA Reductase Dysregulation: Sex Does Matter (A Gender Perspective).* Curr Gerontol Geriatr Res, 2010: p. 420139.

[168] Yasojima, K., E.G. McGeer, and P.L. McGeer, *3-hydroxy-3-methylglutaryl-coenzyme A reductase mRNA in Alzheimer and control brain.* Neuroreport, 2001. 12(13): p. 2935-8.

[169] Eckert, G.P., et al., *Regulation of the brain isoprenoids farnesyl- and geranylgeranylpyrophosphate is altered in male Alzheimer patients.* Neurobiol Dis, 2009. 35(2): p. 251-7.

[170] Do, R., et al., *Squalene synthase: a critical enzyme in the cholesterol biosynthesis pathway.* Clin Genet, 2009. 75(1): p. 19-29.

[171] Tozawa, R., et al., *Embryonic lethality and defective neural tube closure in mice lacking squalene synthase.* J Biol Chem, 1999. 274(43): p. 30843-8.

[172] Lutjohann, D., *Cholesterol metabolism in the brain: importance of 24S-hydroxylation.* Acta Neurol Scand Suppl, 2006. 185: p. 33-42.

[173] Lusa, S., S. Heino, and E. Ikonen, *Differential mobilization of newly synthesized cholesterol and biosynthetic sterol precursors from cells.* J Biol Chem, 2003. 278(22): p. 19844-51.

[174] Johnson, W.J., et al., *Efflux of Newly Synthesized Cholesterol and Biosynthetic Sterol Intermediates from Cells: Dependence on Acceptor Type and on Enrichment of Cells with Cholesterol.* Journal of Biological Chemistry, 1995. 270(42): p. 25037-25046.

[175] Mutka, A.L., et al., *Secretion of sterols and the NPC2 protein from primary astrocytes.* J Biol Chem, 2004. 279(47): p. 48654-62.

[176] Smiljanic, K., et al., *Aging Induces Tissue-Specific Changes in Cholesterol Metabolism in Rat Brain and Liver.* Lipids, 2013.

[177] Lutjohann, D., *Profile of cholesterol-related sterols in aged amyloid precursor protein transgenic mouse brain.* The Journal of Lipid Research, 2002. 43(7): p. 1078-1085.

[178] Tint, G.S., et al., *The use of the Dhcr7 knockout mouse to accurately determine the origin of fetal sterols.* J Lipid Res, 2006. 47(7): p. 1535-41.

[179] Hinse, C.H. and S.N. Shah, *The desmosterol reductase activity of rat brain during development.* J Neurochem, 1971. 18(10): p. 1989-98.

[180] Kritchevsky, D. and W.L. Holmes, *Occurrence of desmosterol in developing rat brain.* Biochem Biophys Res Commun, 1962. 7: p. 128-31.

[181] Fumagalli, R. and R. Paoletti, *The identification and significance of desmosterol in the developing human and animal brain.* Life Sci, 1963. 5: p. 291-5.

[182] Jansen, M., et al., *What dictates the accumulation of desmosterol in the developing brain?* FASEB J, 2013. 27(3): p. 865-70.

[183] Tint, G.S., et al., *Desmosterol in brain is elevated because DHCR24 needs REST for Robust Expression but REST is poorly expressed.* Dev Neurosci, 2014. 36(2): p. 132-42.

[184] Tint, G.S., et al., *The Smith-Lemli-Opitz syndrome: a potentially fatal birth defect caused by a block in the last enzymatic step in cholesterol biosynthesis.* Subcell Biochem, 1997. 28: p. 117-44.

[185] Jira, P., *Cholesterol metabolism deficiency.* Handb Clin Neurol, 2013. 113: p. 1845-50.

[186] Kempen, H.J.M., et al., *Serum Lathosterol Concentration Is an Indicator of Whole-Body Cholesterol-Synthesis in Humans.* Journal of Lipid Research, 1988. 29(9): p. 1149-1155.

[187] Bjorkhem, I., et al., *Correlation between Serum Levels of Some Cholesterol Precursors and Activity of Hmg-Coa Reductase in Human-Liver.* Journal of Lipid Research, 1987. 28(10): p. 1137-1143.

[188] Irons, M., et al., *Defective cholesterol biosynthesis in Smith-Lemli-Opitz syndrome.* Lancet, 1993. 341(8857): p. 1414.

[189] Nowaczyk, M.J. and M.B. Irons, *Smith-Lemli-Opitz syndrome: phenotype, natural history, and epidemiology.* Am J Med Genet C Semin Med Genet, 2012. 160C(4): p. 250-62.

[190] Waterham, H.R., et al., *Mutations in the 3beta-hydroxysterol Delta24-reductase gene cause desmosterolosis, an autosomal recessive disorder of cholesterol biosynthesis.* Am J Hum Genet, 2001. 69(4): p. 685-94.

[191] Belic, A., et al., *An algorithm for rapid computational construction of metabolic networks: a cholesterol biosynthesis example.* Comput Biol Med, 2013. 43(5): p. 471-80.

[192] Bae, S.H. and Y.K. Paik, *Cholesterol biosynthesis from lanosterol: development of a novel assay method and characterization of rat liver microsomal lanosterol delta 24-reductase.* Biochem J, 1997. 326 (Pt 2): p. 609-16.

[193] Wechsler, A., et al., *Generation of viable cholesterol-free mice.* Science, 2003. 302(5653): p. 2087.

[194] FitzPatrick, D.R., et al., *Clinical phenotype of desmosterolosis.* Am J Med Genet, 1998. 75(2): p. 145-52.

[195] Yang, C.D., et al., *Sterol intermediates from cholesterol biosynthetic pathway as liver X receptor ligands.* Journal of Biological Chemistry, 2006. 281(38): p. 27816-27826.

[196] Greeve, I., et al., *The human DIMINUTO/DWARF1 homolog seladin-1 confers resistance to Alzheimer's disease-associated neurodegeneration and oxidative stress.* The Journal of neuroscience : the official journal of the Society for Neuroscience, 2000. 20(19): p. 7345-52.

[197] Luciani, P., et al., *Expression of the antiapoptotic gene seladin-1 and octreotide-induced apoptosis in growth hormone-secreting and nonfunctioning pituitary adenomas.* J Clin Endocrinol Metab, 2005. 90(11): p. 6156-61.

[198] Fuller, P.J., et al., *Seladin-1/DHCR24 expression in normal ovary, ovarian epithelial and granulosa tumours.* Clin Endocrinol (Oxf), 2005. 63(1): p. 111-5.

[199] Biancolella, M., et al., *Effects of dutasteride on the expression of genes related to androgen metabolism and related pathway in human prostate cancer cell lines.* Invest New Drugs, 2007. 25(5): p. 491-7.

[200] Zerenturk, E.J., et al., *Desmosterol and DHCR24: unexpected new directions for a terminal step in cholesterol synthesis.* Prog Lipid Res, 2013. 52(4): p. 666-80.

[201] Nelson, J.A., S.R. Steckbeck, and T.A. Spencer, *Biosynthesis of 24,25-epoxycholesterol from squalene 2,3;22,23-dioxide.* J Biol Chem, 1981. 256(3): p. 1067-8.

[202] Wong, J., C.M. Quinn, and A.J. Brown, *Synthesis of the oxysterol, 24(S), 25-epoxycholesterol, parallels cholesterol production and may protect against cellular accumulation of newly-synthesized cholesterol.* Lipids Health Dis, 2007. 6: p. 10.

[203] Wang, Y., et al., *24S,25-Epoxycholesterol in mouse and rat brain.* Biochem Biophys Res Commun, 2014. 449(2): p. 229-234.

[204] Griffiths, W.J. and Y. Wang, *Analysis of oxysterol metabolomes.* Biochim Biophys Acta, 2011. 1811(11): p. 784-99.

[205] Wong, J., et al., *Endogenous 24(S),25-epoxycholesterol fine-tunes acute control of cellular cholesterol homeostasis.* J Biol Chem, 2008. 283(2): p. 700-7.

[206] Wong, J., et al., *Primary human astrocytes produce 24(S),25-epoxycholesterol with implications for brain cholesterol homeostasis.* J Neurochem, 2007. 103(5): p. 1764-73.

[207] Janowski, B.A., et al., *Structural requirements of ligands for the oxysterol liver X receptors LXRalpha and LXRbeta.* Proc Natl Acad Sci U S A, 1999. 96(1): p. 266-71.

[208] Beyea, M.M., et al., *Selective up-regulation of LXR-regulated genes ABCA1, ABCG1, and APOE in macrophages through increased endogenous synthesis of 24(S),25-epoxycholesterol.* J Biol Chem, 2007. 282(8): p. 5207-16.

[209] Horton, J.D., *Sterol regulatory element-binding proteins: transcriptional activators of lipid synthesis.* Biochem Soc Trans, 2002. 30(Pt 6): p. 1091-5.

[210] Gill, S., et al., *Cholesterol-dependent degradation of squalene monooxygenase, a control point in cholesterol synthesis beyond HMG-CoA reductase.* Cell Metab, 2011. 13(3): p. 260-73.

[211] Foresti, O., et al., *Sterol homeostasis requires regulated degradation of squalene monooxygenase by the ubiquitin ligase Doa10/Teb4.* Elife, 2013. 2: p. e00953.

[212] Daimiel, L.A., et al., *Promoter analysis of the DHCR24 (3beta-hydroxysterol Delta(24)-reductase) gene: characterization of SREBP (sterol-regulatory-element-binding protein)-mediated activation.* Biosci Rep, 2013. 33(1): p. 57-69.

[213] Demoulin, J.B., et al., *Platelet-derived growth factor stimulates membrane lipid synthesis through activation of phosphatidylinositol 3-kinase and sterol regulatory element-binding proteins.* J Biol Chem, 2004. 279(34): p. 35392-402.

[214] Reed, B.D., et al., *Genome-wide occupancy of SREBP1 and its partners NFY and SP1 reveals novel functional roles and combinatorial regulation of distinct classes of genes.* PLoS Genet, 2008. 4(7): p. e1000133.

[215] Ramos, M.C., et al., *Simvastatin modulates the Alzheimer's disease-related gene seladin-1.* J Alzheimers Dis, 2012. 28(2): p. 297-301.

[216] Wang, Y., et al., *The selective Alzheimer's disease indicator-1 gene (Seladin-1/DHCR24) is a liver X receptor target gene.* Molecular pharmacology, 2008. 74(6): p. 1716-21.

[217] Drzewinska, J., A. Walczak-Drzewiecka, and M. Ratajewski, *Identification and analysis of the promoter region of the human DHCR24 gene: involvement of DNA methylation and histone acetylation.* Mol Biol Rep, 2011. 38(2): p. 1091-101.

[218] Zerenturk, E.J., et al., *The endogenous regulator 24(S),25-epoxycholesterol inhibits cholesterol synthesis at DHCR24 (Seladin-1).* Biochim Biophys Acta, 2012. 1821(9): p. 1269-77.

[219] Luu, W., et al., *Signaling regulates activity of DHCR24, the final enzyme in cholesterol synthesis.* J Lipid Res, 2014. 55(3): p. 410-20.

[220] Iivonen, S., et al., *Seladin-1 transcription is linked to neuronal degeneration in Alzheimer's disease.* Neuroscience, 2002. 113(2): p. 301-10.

[221] Sharpe, L.J., et al., *Is seladin-1 really a selective Alzheimer's disease indicator?* J Alzheimers Dis, 2012. 30(1): p. 35-9.

[222] Lamsa, R., et al., *The association study between DHCR24 polymorphisms and Alzheimer's disease*. Am J Med Genet B Neuropsychiatr Genet, 2007. 144B(7): p. 906-10.

[223] Feher, A., et al., *Gender dependent effect of DHCR24 polymorphism on the risk for Alzheimer's disease*. Neurosci Lett, 2012. 526(1): p. 20-3.

[224] Benvenuti, S., et al., *Neuronal differentiation of human mesenchymal stem cells: changes in the expression of the Alzheimer's disease-related gene seladin-1*. Exp Cell Res, 2006. 312(13): p. 2592-604.

[225] Peri, A., et al., *New insights on the neuroprotective role of sterols and sex steroids: the seladin-1/DHCR24 paradigm*. Front Neuroendocrinol, 2009. 30(2): p. 119-29.

[226] Lu, T., et al., *REST and stress resistance in ageing and Alzheimer's disease*. Nature, 2014. 507(7493): p. 448-54.

[227] Wisniewski, T., K. Newman, and N.B. Javitt, *Alzheimer's disease: brain desmosterol levels*. J Alzheimers Dis, 2013. 33(3): p. 881-8.

[228] Peri, A. and M. Serio, *Neuroprotective effects of the Alzheimer's disease-related gene seladin-1*. J Mol Endocrinol, 2008. 41(5): p. 251-61.

[229] Lu, X., et al., *3 beta-hydroxysteroid-Delta 24 reductase (DHCR24) protects neuronal cells from apoptotic cell death induced by endoplasmic reticulum (ER) stress*. PLoS One, 2014. 9(1): p. e86753.

[230] Luciani, P., et al., *Seladin-1 is a fundamental mediator of the neuroprotective effects of estrogen in human neuroblast long-term cell cultures*. Endocrinology, 2008. 149(9): p. 4256-66.

[231] Benvenuti, S., et al., *Estrogen and selective estrogen receptor modulators exert neuroprotective effects and stimulate the expression of selective Alzheimer's disease indicator-1, a recently discovered antiapoptotic gene, in human neuroblast long-term cell cultures*. J Clin Endocrinol Metab, 2005. 90(3): p. 1775-82.

[232] Peri, A., et al., *Membrane cholesterol as a mediator of the neuroprotective effects of estrogens*. Neuroscience, 2011. 191: p. 107-17.

[233] Cecchi, C., et al., *Seladin-1/DHCR24 protects neuroblastoma cells against Abeta toxicity by increasing membrane cholesterol content*. Journal of cellular and molecular medicine, 2008. 12(5B): p. 1990-2002.

[234] Pensalfini, A., et al., *Membrane cholesterol enrichment prevents Abeta-induced oxidative stress in Alzheimer's fibroblasts*. Neurobiol Aging, 2011. 32(2): p. 210-22.

[235] Crameri, A., et al., *The role of seladin-1/DHCR24 in cholesterol biosynthesis, APP processing and Abeta generation in vivo*. EMBO J, 2006. 25(2): p. 432-43.

[236] Martin, M., C.G. Dotti, and M.D. Ledesma, *Brain cholesterol in normal and pathological aging*. Biochim Biophys Acta, 2010. 1801(8): p. 934-944.

[237] Cossec, J.C., et al., *Cholesterol changes in Alzheimer's disease: Methods of analysis and impact on the formation of enlarged endosomes.* Biochim Biophys Acta, 2010.

[238] Wood, W.G., et al., *Cholesterol as a causative factor in Alzheimer's disease: a debatable hypothesis.* J Neurochem, 2014. 129(4): p. 559-72.

[239] Edlund, C., et al., *Ubiquinone, dolichol, and cholesterol metabolism in aging and Alzheimer's disease.* Biochemistry and cell biology = Biochimie et biologie cellulaire, 1992. 70(6): p. 422-8.

[240] Snipes, G.J. and U. Suter, *Cholesterol and myelin.* Subcell Biochem, 1997. 28: p. 173-204.

[241] Eckert, G.P., et al., *Cholesterol modulates the membrane-disordering effects of beta-amyloid peptides in the hippocampus: specific changes in Alzheimer's disease.* Dement Geriatr Cogn Disord, 2000. 11(4): p. 181-6.

[242] Heverin, M., et al., *Changes in the levels of cerebral and extracerebral sterols in the brain of patients with Alzheimer's disease.* J Lipid Res, 2004. 45(1): p. 186-93.

[243] Cutler, R.G., et al., *Involvement of oxidative stress-induced abnormalities in ceramide and cholesterol metabolism in brain aging and Alzheimer's disease.* Proc Natl Acad Sci U S A, 2004. 101(7): p. 2070-5.

[244] Mori, T., et al., *Cholesterol accumulates in senile plaques of Alzheimer disease patients and in transgenic APP(SW) mice.* J Neuropathol Exp Neurol, 2001. 60(8): p. 778-85.

[245] Panchal, M., et al., *Enrichment of cholesterol in microdissected Alzheimer's disease senile plaques as assessed by mass spectrometry.* J Lipid Res, 2010. 51(3): p. 598-605.

[246] Mason, R.P., et al., *Evidence for changes in the Alzheimer's disease brain cortical membrane structure mediated by cholesterol.* Neurobiol Aging, 1992. 13(3): p. 413-9.

[247] Hascalovici, J.R., et al., *Brain sterol dysregulation in sporadic AD and MCI: relationship to heme oxygenase-1.* J Neurochem, 2009. 110(4): p. 1241-53.

[248] Kolsch, H., et al., *Alterations of cholesterol precursor levels in Alzheimer's disease.* Biochim Biophys Acta, 2010. 1801(8): p. 945-50.

[249] Mulder, M., et al., *Reduced levels of cholesterol, phospholipids, and fatty acids in cerebrospinal fluid of Alzheimer disease patients are not related to apolipoprotein E4.* Alzheimer Dis Assoc Disord, 1998. 12(3): p. 198-203.

[250] Wender, M., Z. Adamczewska-Goncerzewicz, and J. Szczech, *Free sterols in senile human brain.* Folia Neuropathol, 1994. 32(2): p. 75-9.

[251] Naylor, J.C., et al., *Allopregnanolone levels are reduced in temporal cortex in patients with Alzheimer's disease compared to cognitively intact control subjects.* Biochim Biophys Acta, 2010. 1801(8): p. 951-9.

[252] Burns, M. and K. Duff, *Cholesterol in Alzheimer's disease and tauopathy.* Annals of the New York Academy of Sciences, 2002. 977: p. 367-75.

[253] Lazar, A.N., et al., *Time-of-flight secondary ion mass spectrometry (TOF-SIMS) imaging reveals cholesterol overload in the cerebral cortex of Alzheimer disease patients.* Acta Neuropathol, 2013. 125(1): p. 133-44.

[254] Ohm, T.G., et al., *Cholesterol and tau protein--findings in Alzheimer's and Niemann Pick C's disease.* Pharmacopsychiatry, 2003. 36 Suppl 2: p. S120-6.

[255] Gomez-Ramos, P. and M. Asuncion Moran, *Ultrastructural localization of intraneuronal Abeta-peptide in Alzheimer disease brains.* J Alzheimers Dis, 2007. 11(1): p. 53-9.

[256] Fernandez, A., et al., *Mitochondrial cholesterol loading exacerbates amyloid beta peptide-induced inflammation and neurotoxicity.* J Neurosci, 2009. 29(20): p. 6394-405.

[257] Sole-Domenech, S., et al., *Localization of cholesterol, amyloid and glia in Alzheimer's disease transgenic mouse brain tissue using time-of-flight secondary ion mass spectrometry (ToF-SIMS) and immunofluorescence imaging.* Acta Neuropathol, 2013. 125(1): p. 145-57.

[258] Aqul, A., et al., *Unesterified cholesterol accumulation in late endosomes/lysosomes causes neurodegeneration and is prevented by driving cholesterol export from this compartment.* J Neurosci, 2011. 31(25): p. 9404-13.

[259] Yamazaki, T., et al., *Accumulation and aggregation of amyloid beta-protein in late endosomes of Niemann-pick type C cells.* J Biol Chem, 2001. 276(6): p. 4454-60.

[260] Auer, I.A., et al., *Paired helical filament tau (PHFtau) in Niemann-Pick type C disease is similar to PHFtau in Alzheimer's disease.* Acta Neuropathol (Berl), 1995. 90(6): p. 547-51.

[261] Saito, Y., et al., *Niemann-Pick type C disease: accelerated neurofibrillary tangle formation and amyloid beta deposition associated with apolipoprotein E epsilon 4 homozygosity.* Ann Neurol, 2002. 52(3): p. 351-5.

[262] Nixon, R.A., *Niemann-Pick Type C disease and Alzheimer's disease: the APP-endosome connection fattens up.* Am J Pathol, 2004. 164(3): p. 757-61.

[263] Jin, L.W., et al., *Intracellular accumulation of amyloidogenic fragments of amyloid-beta precursor protein in neurons with Niemann-Pick type C defects is associated with endosomal abnormalities.* Am J Pathol, 2004. 164(3): p. 975-85.

[264] Yao, J., et al., *Neuroprotection by cyclodextrin in cell and mouse models of Alzheimer disease.* J Exp Med, 2012. 209(13): p. 2501-13.

[265] Hudry, E., et al., *Adeno-associated virus gene therapy with cholesterol 24-hydroxylase reduces the amyloid pathology before or after the onset of amyloid plaques in mouse models of Alzheimer's disease.* Molecular therapy : the journal of the American Society of Gene Therapy, 2010. 18(1): p. 44-53.

[266] Bu, G., *Apolipoprotein E and its receptors in Alzheimer's disease: pathways, pathogenesis and therapy.* Nat Rev Neurosci, 2009. 10(5): p. 333-44.

[267] Verghese, P.B., J.M. Castellano, and D.M. Holtzman, *Apolipoprotein E in Alzheimer's disease and other neurological disorders.* Lancet Neurol, 2011. 10(3): p. 241-52.

[268] Grimm, M.O., et al., *The impact of cholesterol, DHA, and sphingolipids on Alzheimer's disease.* Biomed Res Int, 2013. 2013: p. 814390.

[269] Fonseca, A.C., et al., *Cholesterol and statins in Alzheimer's disease: current controversies.* Exp Neurol, 2010. 223(2): p. 282-93.

[270] Pfrieger, F.W., *Role of cholesterol in synapse formation and function.* Biochim Biophys Acta, 2003. 1610(2): p. 271-80.

[271] Dotti, C.G., J.A. Esteban, and M.D. Ledesma, *Lipid dynamics at dendritic spines.* Front Neuroanat, 2014. 8: p. 76.

[272] Selkoe, D.J., *Alzheimer's disease is a synaptic failure.* Science, 2002. 298(5594): p. 789-91.

[273] Tanzi, R.E., *The synaptic Abeta hypothesis of Alzheimer disease.* Nat Neurosci, 2005. 8(8): p. 977-9.

[274] Ferrer, I. and F. Gullotta, *Down's syndrome and Alzheimer's disease: dendritic spine counts in the hippocampus.* Acta Neuropathol, 1990. 79(6): p. 680-5.

[275] Moolman, D.L., et al., *Dendrite and dendritic spine alterations in Alzheimer models.* J Neurocytol, 2004. 33(3): p. 377-87.

[276] Spires, T.L., et al., *Dendritic spine abnormalities in amyloid precursor protein transgenic mice demonstrated by gene transfer and intravital multiphoton microscopy.* J Neurosci, 2005. 25(31): p. 7278-87.

[277] Jacobsen, J.S., et al., *Early-onset behavioral and synaptic deficits in a mouse model of Alzheimer's disease.* Proc Natl Acad Sci U S A, 2006. 103(13): p. 5161-6.

[278] Knafo, S., et al., *Widespread changes in dendritic spines in a model of Alzheimer's disease.* Cereb Cortex, 2009. 19(3): p. 586-92.

[279] Koudinov, A.R. and N.V. Koudinova, *Cholesterol homeostasis failure as a unifying cause of synaptic degeneration.* J Neurol Sci, 2005. 229-230: p. 233-40.

[280] Rajanikant, G.K., et al., *The therapeutic potential of statins in neurological disorders.* Curr Med Chem, 2007. 14(1): p. 103-12.

[281] Obiol-Pardo, C., J. Rubio-Martinez, and S. Imperial, *The Methylerythritol Phosphate (MEP) Pathway for Isoprenoid Biosynthesis as a Target for the Development of New Drugs Against Tuberculosis.* Current Medicinal Chemistry, 2011. 18(9): p. 1325-1338.

[282] Wiemer, A.J., R.J. Hohl, and D.F. Wiemer, *The Intermediate Enzymes of Isoprenoid Metabolism as Anticancer Targets.* Anti-Cancer Agents in Medicinal Chemistry, 2009. 9(5): p. 526-542.

[283] Kandutsch, A.A., et al., *Purification of Geranylgeranyl Pyrophosphate Synthetase from Micrococcus Lysodeikticus.* J Biol Chem, 1964. 239: p. 2507-15.

[284] Ericsson, J., et al., *Distribution of prenyltransferases in rat tissues. Evidence for a cytosolic all-trans-geranylgeranyl diphosphate synthase.* J Biol Chem, 1993. 268(2): p. 832-8.

[285] Runquist, M., et al., *Distribution of branch point prenyltransferases in regions of bovine brain.* J Neurochem, 1995. 65(5): p. 2299-306.

[286] Park, J., et al., *Human isoprenoid synthase enzymes as therapeutic targets.* Front Chem, 2014. 2: p. 50.

[287] Afshordel, S., et al., *Impaired geranylgeranyltransferase-I regulation reduces membrane-associated Rho protein levels in aged mouse brain.* J Neurochem, 2014. 129(4): p. 732-42.

[288] Schenk, B., F. Fernandez, and C.J. Waechter, *The ins(ide) and out(side) of dolichyl phosphate biosynthesis and recycling in the endoplasmic reticulum.* Glycobiology, 2001. 11(5): p. 61R-70R.

[289] Crick, D.C., J.S. Rush, and C.J. Waechter, *Characterization and localization of a long-chain isoprenyltransferase activity in porcine brain: proposed role in the biosynthesis of dolichyl phosphate.* J Neurochem, 1991. 57(4): p. 1354-62.

[290] Takeda, J. and T. Kinoshita, *GPI-anchor biosynthesis.* Trends Biochem Sci, 1995. 20(9): p. 367-71.

[291] Kornfeld, R. and S. Kornfeld, *Assembly of asparagine-linked oligosaccharides.* Annu Rev Biochem, 1985. 54: p. 631-64.

[292] Andersson, M., et al., *Age-dependent changes in the levels of dolichol and dolichyl phosphates in human brain.* Acta Chem Scand B, 1987. 41(2): p. 144-6.

[293] Pallottini, V., et al., *Age-related changes of isoprenoid biosynthesis in rat liver and brain.* Biogerontology, 2003. 4(6): p. 371-8.

[294] Parentini, I., et al., *Accumulation of dolichol in older tissues satisfies the proposed criteria to be qualified a biomarker of aging.* J Gerontol A Biol Sci Med Sci, 2005. 60(1): p. 39-43.

[295] Dallner, G. and P.J. Sindelar, *Regulation of ubiquinone metabolism.* Free Radic Biol Med, 2000. 29(3-4): p. 285-94.

[296] Teclebrhan, H., et al., *Biosynthesis of the side chain of ubiquinone:trans-prenyltransferase in rat liver microsomes.* J Biol Chem, 1993. 268(31): p. 23081-6.

[297] Rauthan, M. and M. Pilon, *The mevalonate pathway in C. elegans.* Lipids Health Dis, 2011. 10: p. 243.

[298] Lopez-Lluch, G., et al., *Is coenzyme Q a key factor in aging?* Mech Ageing Dev, 2010. 131(4): p. 225-35.

[299] Bentinger, M., et al., *Distribution and breakdown of labeled coenzyme Q10 in rat.* Free Radic Biol Med, 2003. 34(5): p. 563-75.

[300] Bansal, V.S. and S. Vaidya, *Characterization of two distinct allyl pyrophosphatase activities from rat liver microsomes.* Arch Biochem Biophys, 1994. 315(2): p. 393-9.

[301] Miriyala, S., et al., *Functional characterization of the atypical integral membrane lipid phosphatase PDP1/PPAPDC2 identifies a pathway for interconversion of isoprenols and isoprenoid phosphates in mammalian cells.* J Biol Chem, 2010. 285(18): p. 13918-29.

[302] Crick, D.C., D.A. Andres, and C.J. Waechter, *Novel salvage pathway utilizing farnesol and geranylgeraniol for protein isoprenylation.* Biochem Biophys Res Commun, 1997. 237(3): p. 483-7.

[303] Beigneux, A., et al., *Prenylcysteine lyase deficiency in mice results in the accumulation of farnesylcysteine and geranylgeranylcysteine in brain and liver.* J Biol Chem, 2002. 277(41): p. 38358-63.

[304] Onono, F., et al., *Efficient use of exogenous isoprenols for protein isoprenylation by MDA-MB-231 cells is regulated independently of the mevalonate pathway.* J Biol Chem, 2013. 288(38): p. 27444-55.

[305] Crick, D.C., C.J. Waechter, and D.A. Andres, *Utilization of geranylgeraniol for protein isoprenylation in C6 glial cells.* Biochem Biophys Res Commun, 1994. 205(1): p. 955-61.

[306] Ownby, S.E. and R.J. Hohl, *Isoprenoid alcohols restore protein isoprenylation in a time-dependent manner independent of protein synthesis.* Lipids, 2003. 38(7): p. 751-9.

[307] Fernandes, N.V., et al., *Geranylgeraniol suppresses the viability of human DU145 prostate carcinoma cells and the level of HMG CoA reductase.* Exp Biol Med (Maywood), 2013. 238(11): p. 1265-74.

[308] Roullet, J.B., et al., *Modulation of neuronal voltage-gated calcium channels by farnesol.* J Biol Chem, 1999. 274(36): p. 25439-46.

[309] Forman, B.M., et al., *Identification of a nuclear receptor that is activated by farnesol metabolites.* Cell, 1995. 81(5): p. 687-93.

[310] Sebti, S.M., *Protein farnesylation: implications for normal physiology, malignant transformation, and cancer therapy.* Cancer Cell, 2005. 7(4): p. 297-300.

[311] McTaggart, S.J., *Isoprenylated proteins.* Cell Mol Life Sci, 2006. 63(3): p. 255-67.

[312] Bento, C.F., et al., *The role of membrane-trafficking small GTPases in the regulation of autophagy.* J Cell Sci, 2013. 126(Pt 5): p. 1059-69.

[313] Wiemer, A.J., D.F. Wiemer, and R.J. Hohl, *Geranylgeranyl diphosphate synthase: an emerging therapeutic target.* Clin Pharmacol Ther, 2011. 90(6): p. 804-12.

[314] Lane, K.T. and L.S. Beese, *Thematic review series: lipid posttranslational modifications. Structural biology of protein farnesyltransferase and geranylgeranyltransferase type I.* J Lipid Res, 2006. 47(4): p. 681-99.

[315] Leung, K.F., R. Baron, and M.C. Seabra, *Thematic review series: lipid posttranslational modifications. geranylgeranylation of Rab GTPases.* J Lipid Res, 2006. 47(3): p. 467-75.

[316] Desnoyers, L., J.S. Anant, and M.C. Seabra, *Geranylgeranylation of Rab proteins.* Biochem Soc Trans, 1996. 24(3): p. 699-703.

[317] Wu, S.K., et al., *Structural insights into the function of the Rab GDI superfamily.* Trends Biochem Sci, 1996. 21(12): p. 472-6.

[318] Seabra, M.C., et al., *Rab geranylgeranyl transferase. A multisubunit enzyme that prenylates GTP-binding proteins terminating in Cys-X-Cys or Cys-Cys.* J Biol Chem, 1992. 267(20): p. 14497-503.

[319] Farnsworth, C.C., et al., *Rab geranylgeranyl transferase catalyzes the geranylgeranylation of adjacent cysteines in the small GTPases Rab1A, Rab3A, and Rab5A.* Proc Natl Acad Sci U S A, 1994. 91(25): p. 11963-7.

[320] Gomes, A.Q., et al., *Membrane targeting of Rab GTPases is influenced by the prenylation motif.* Mol Biol Cell, 2003. 14(5): p. 1882-99.

[321] Holstein, S.A. and R.J. Hohl, *Is there a future for prenyltransferase inhibitors in cancer therapy?* Curr Opin Pharmacol, 2012. 12(6): p. 704-9.

[322] Gelb, M.H., et al., *Therapeutic intervention based on protein prenylation and associated modifications.* Nat Chem Biol, 2006. 2(10): p. 518-28.

[323] Lebowitz, P.F., W. Du, and G.C. Prendergast, *Prenylation of RhoB is required for its cell transforming function but not its ability to activate serum response element-dependent transcription.* J Biol Chem, 1997. 272(26): p. 16093-5.

[324] Allal, C., et al., *RhoA prenylation is required for promotion of cell growth and transformation and cytoskeleton organization but not for induction of serum response element transcription.* J Biol Chem, 2000. 275(40): p. 31001-8.

[325] Miyake, M., et al., *Unfarnesylated transforming Ras mutant inhibits the Ras-signaling pathway by forming a stable Ras.Raf complex in the cytosol.* FEBS Lett, 1996. 378(1): p. 15-8.

[326] Ntantie, E., et al., *An Adenosine-Mediated Signaling Pathway Suppresses Prenylation of the GTPase Rap1B and Promotes Cell Scattering.* Science Signaling, 2013. 6(277): p. ra39-ra39.

[327] Khan, O.M., et al., *Geranylgeranyltransferase type I (GGTase-I) deficiency hyperactivates macrophages and induces erosive arthritis in mice.* J Clin Invest, 2011. 121(2): p. 628-39.

[328] Konstantinopoulos, P.A., M.V. Karamouzis, and A.G. Papavassiliou, *Post-translational modifications and regulation of the RAS superfamily of GTPases as anticancer targets.* Nat Rev Drug Discov, 2007. 6(7): p. 541-55.

[329] Li, L., et al., *Isoprenoids and Related Pharmacological Interventions: Potential Application in Alzheimer's Disease.* Mol Neurobiol, 2012.

[330] Cole, S.L. and R. Vassar, *Isoprenoids and Alzheimer's disease: a complex relationship.* Neurobiol Dis, 2006. 22(2): p. 209-22.

[331] Butterfield, D.A., E. Barone, and C. Mancuso, *Cholesterol-independent neuroprotective and neurotoxic activities of statins: perspectives for statin use in Alzheimer disease and other age-related neurodegenerative disorders.* Pharmacological research : the official journal of the Italian Pharmacological Society, 2011. 64(3): p. 180-6.

[332] van der Most, P.J., et al., *Statins: mechanisms of neuroprotection.* Prog Neurobiol, 2009. 88(1): p. 64-75.

[333] Wood, W.G., et al., *Statins and neuroprotection: a prescription to move the field forward.* Ann N Y Acad Sci, 2010. 1199: p. 69-76.

[334] Liao, J.K., *Isoprenoids as mediators of the biological effects of statins.* J Clin Invest, 2002. 110(3): p. 285-8.

[335] Luo, Z.G., et al., *Implication of geranylgeranyltransferase I in synapse formation.* Neuron, 2003. 40(4): p. 703-17.

[336] Joly, A., G. Popjak, and P.A. Edwards, *In vitro identification of a soluble protein:geranylgeranyl transferase from rat tissues.* J Biol Chem, 1991. 266(21): p. 13495-8.

[337] Zhou, X.P., et al., *TrkB-mediated activation of geranylgeranyltransferase I promotes dendritic morphogenesis.* Proc Natl Acad Sci U S A, 2008. 105(44): p. 17181-6.

[338] Li, Z., et al., *Geranylgeranyltransferase I mediates BDNF-induced synaptogenesis.* J Neurochem, 2013. 125(5): p. 698-712.

[339] Wu, K.Y., X.P. Zhou, and Z.G. Luo, *Geranylgeranyltransferase I is essential for dendritic development of cerebellar Purkinje cells.* Mol Brain, 2010. 3: p. 18.

[340] Wood, W.G., W.E. Mupsilonller, and G.P. Eckert, *Statins and Neuroprotection: Basic Pharmacology Needed.* Mol Neurobiol, 2014.

[341] Pooler, A.M., S.C. Xi, and R.J. Wurtman, *The 3-hydroxy-3-methylglutaryl co-enzyme A reductase inhibitor pravastatin enhances neurite outgrowth in hippocampal neurons.* Journal of neurochemistry, 2006. 97(3): p. 716-23.

[342] Maltese, W.A. and K.M. Sheridan, *Differentiation of neuroblastoma cells induced by an inhibitor of mevalonate synthesis: relation of neurite outgrowth and acetylcholinesterase activity to changes in cell proliferation and blocked isoprenoid synthesis.* J Cell Physiol, 1985. 125(3): p. 540-58.

[343] Fernandez-Hernando, C., Y. Suarez, and M.A. Lasuncion, *Lovastatin-induced PC-12 cell differentiation is associated with RhoA/RhoA kinase pathway inactivation.* Molecular and cellular neurosciences, 2005. 29(4): p. 591-602.

[344] Holmberg, E., et al., *Simvastatin promotes neurite outgrowth in the presence of inhibitory molecules found in central nervous system injury.* J Neurotrauma, 2006. 23(9): p. 1366-78.

[345] Schulz, J.G., et al., *HMG-CoA reductase inhibition causes neurite loss by interfering with geranylgeranylpyrophosphate synthesis.* Journal of neurochemistry, 2004. 89(1): p. 24-32.

[346] Kim, W.Y., et al., *Statins decrease dendritic arborization in rat sympathetic neurons by blocking RhoA activation.* J Neurochem, 2009. 108(4): p. 1057-71.

[347] de Chaves, E.I., et al., *Role of lipoproteins in the delivery of lipids to axons during axonal regeneration.* J Biol Chem, 1997. 272(49): p. 30766-73.

[348] Samuel, F., et al., *Inhibiting geranylgeranylation increases neurite branching and differentially activates cofilin in cell bodies and growth cones.* Mol Neurobiol, 2014. 50(1): p. 49-59.

[349] Garcia-Roman, N., et al., *Lovastatin induces apoptosis of spontaneously immortalized rat brain neuroblasts: involvement of nonsterol isoprenoid biosynthesis inhibition.* Molecular and cellular neurosciences, 2001. 17(2): p. 329-41.

[350] Saavedra, L., et al., *Internalization of beta-amyloid peptide by primary neurons in the absence of apolipoprotein E.* J Biol Chem, 2007. 282(49): p. 35722-32.

[351] Marz, P., U. Otten, and A.R. Miserez, *Statins induce differentiation and cell death in neurons and astroglia.* Glia, 2007. 55(1): p. 1-12.

[352] Bi, X.N., et al., *Inhibition of geranylgeranylation mediates the effects of 3-hydroxy-3-methylglutaryl (HMG)-CoA reductase inhibitors on microglia.* Journal of Biological Chemistry, 2004. 279(46): p. 48238-48245.

[353] Naidu, A., et al., *Secretion of apolipoprotein E by brain glia requires protein prenylation and is suppressed by statins.* Brain Res, 2002. 958(1): p. 100-11.

[354] Bliss, T.V. and G.L. Collingridge, *A synaptic model of memory: long-term potentiation in the hippocampus.* Nature, 1993. 361(6407): p. 31-9.

[355] Kotti, T., et al., *Biphasic requirement for geranylgeraniol in hippocampal long-term potentiation.* Proceedings of the National Academy of Sciences of the United States of America, 2008. 105(32): p. 11394-9.

[356] Mans, R.A., L.L. McMahon, and L. Li, *Simvastatin-mediated enhancement of long-term potentiation is driven by farnesyl-pyrophosphate depletion and inhibition of farnesylation.* Neuroscience, 2012. 202: p. 1-9.

[357]   Posada-Duque, R.A., et al., *Atorvastatin requires geranylgeranyl transferase-I and Rac1 activation to exert neuronal protection and induce plasticity.* Neurochem Int, 2013. 62(4): p. 433-445.

[358]   Samuel, F. and D.L. Hynds, *RHO GTPase signaling for axon extension: is prenylation important?* Molecular neurobiology, 2010. 42(2): p. 133-42.

[359]   Roberts, P.J., et al., *Rho Family GTPase modification and dependence on CAAX motif-signaled posttranslational modification.* J Biol Chem, 2008. 283(37): p. 25150-63.

[360]   Ramakers, G.J., *Rho proteins, mental retardation and the cellular basis of cognition.* Trends Neurosci, 2002. 25(4): p. 191-9.

[361]   Tolias, K.F., J.G. Duman, and K. Um, *Control of synapse development and plasticity by Rho GTPase regulatory proteins.* Prog Neurobiol, 2011. 94(2): p. 133-48.

[362]   DeGeer, J. and N. Lamarche-Vane, *Rho GTPases in neurodegeneration diseases.* Exp Cell Res, 2013. 319(15): p. 2384-94.

[363]   Garcia-Mata, R., E. Boulter, and K. Burridge, *The 'invisible hand': regulation of RHO GTPases by RHOGDIs.* Nature reviews. Molecular cell biology, 2011. 12(8): p. 493-504.

[364]   Medina, M.W., et al., *RHOA is a modulator of the cholesterol-lowering effects of statin.* PLoS Genet, 2012. 8(11): p. e1003058.

[365]   Holstein, S.A., C.L. Wohlford-Lenane, and R.J. Hohl, *Consequences of mevalonate depletion. Differential transcriptional, translational, and post-translational up-regulation of Ras, Rap1a, RhoA, AND RhoB.* J Biol Chem, 2002. 277(12): p. 10678-82.

[366]   Dimster-Denk, D., W.R. Schafer, and J. Rine, *Control of RAS mRNA level by the mevalonate pathway.* Mol Biol Cell, 1995. 6(1): p. 59-70.

[367]   Stubbs, E.B., Jr. and C.L. Von Zee, *Prenylation of Rho G-proteins: a novel mechanism regulating gene expression and protein stability in human trabecular meshwork cells.* Mol Neurobiol, 2012. 46(1): p. 28-40.

[368]   Laezza, C., et al., *Control of Rab5 and Rab7 expression by the isoprenoid pathway.* Biochem Biophys Res Commun, 1998. 248(3): p. 469-72.

[369]   Bifulco, M., *Role of the isoprenoid pathway in ras transforming activity, cytoskeleton organization, cell proliferation and apoptosis.* Life Sci, 2005. 77(14): p. 1740-9.

[370]   Holstein, S.A., C.L. Wohlford-Lenane, and R.J. Hohl, *Isoprenoids influence expression of Ras and Ras-related proteins.* Biochemistry, 2002. 41(46): p. 13698-704.

[371]   Ericsson, J., et al., *Sterol regulatory element binding protein binds to a cis element in the promoter of the farnesyl diphosphate synthase gene.* Proceedings of the National Academy of Sciences of the United States of America, 1996. 93(2): p. 945-950.

[372]   Fukuchi, J., et al., *Transcriptional regulation of farnesyl pyrophosphate synthase by liver X receptors.* Steroids, 2003. 68(7-8): p. 685-691.

[373] Lutz, R.J., T.M. McLain, and M. Sinensky, *Feedback inhibition of polyisoprenyl pyrophosphate synthesis from mevalonate in vitro. Implications for protein prenylation.* J Biol Chem, 1992. 267(12): p. 7983-6.

[374] Laskovics, F.M., J.M. Krafcik, and C.D. Poulter, *Prenyltransferase. Kinetic studies of the 1'-4 coupling reaction with avian liver enzyme.* J Biol Chem, 1979. 254(19): p. 9458-63.

[375] Ericsson, J., et al., *Human geranylgeranyl diphosphate synthase: isolation of the cDNA, chromosomal mapping and tissue expression.* J Lipid Res, 1998. 39(9): p. 1731-9.

[376] Shimano, H., *Sterol regulatory element-binding proteins (SREBPs): transcriptional regulators of lipid synthetic genes.* Progress in lipid research, 2001. 40(6): p. 439-52.

[377] Kavanagh, K.L., et al., *The crystal structure of human geranylgeranyl pyrophosphate synthase reveals a novel hexameric arrangement and inhibitory product binding.* J Biol Chem, 2006. 281(31): p. 22004-12.

[378] Wiemer, A.J., et al., *Digeranyl bisphosphonate inhibits geranylgeranyl pyrophosphate synthase.* Biochem Biophys Res Commun, 2007. 353(4): p. 921-5.

[379] Vicent, D., E. Maratos-Flier, and C.R. Kahn, *The branch point enzyme of the mevalonate pathway for protein prenylation is overexpressed in the ob/ob mouse and induced by adipogenesis.* Mol Cell Biol, 2000. 20(6): p. 2158-66.

[380] Biller, S.A., et al., *Isoprenoid (Phosphinylmethyl)Phosphonates as Inhibitors of Squalene Synthetase.* Journal of Medicinal Chemistry, 1988. 31(10): p. 1869-1871.

[381] James, M.J. and A.A. Kandutsch, *Regulation of hepatic dolichol synthesis by beta-hydroxy-beta-methylglutaryl coenzyme A reductase.* J Biol Chem, 1980. 255(18): p. 8618-22.

[382] Gold, P.H. and R.E. Olson, *Studies on coenzyme Q. The biosynthesis of coenzyme Q9 in rat tissue slices.* J Biol Chem, 1966. 241(15): p. 3507-16.

[383] Sinensky, M., et al., *Differential inhibitory effects of lovastatin on protein isoprenylation and sterol synthesis.* J Biol Chem, 1990. 265(32): p. 19937-41.

[384] Winter-Vann, A.M. and P.J. Casey, *Opinion - Post-prenylation-processing enzymes as new targets in oncogenesis.* Nature Reviews Cancer, 2005. 5(5): p. 405-412.

[385] Edlund, C., M. Soderberg, and K. Kristensson, *Isoprenoids in aging and neurodegeneration.* Neurochem Int, 1994. 25(1): p. 35-8.

[386] Soderberg, M., et al., *Lipid compositions of different regions of the human brain during aging.* J Neurochem, 1990. 54(2): p. 415-23.

[387] Andersson, M., et al., *Age-dependent modifications in the metabolism of mevalonate pathway lipids in rat brain.* Mech Ageing Dev, 1995. 85(1): p. 1-14.

[388] Zhang, Y., et al., *The lipid compositions of different regions of rat brain during development and aging.* Neurobiol Aging, 1996. 17(6): p. 869-75.

[389] Hooff, G.P., et al., *Modulation of cholesterol, farnesylpyrophosphate, and geranylgeranyl-pyrophosphate in neuroblastoma SH-SY5Y-APP695 cells: impact on amyloid beta-protein production*. Molecular neurobiology, 2010. 41(2-3): p. 341-50.

[390] Pedrini, S., et al., *Modulation of statin-activated shedding of Alzheimer APP ectodomain by ROCK*. PLoS Med, 2005. 2(1): p. e18.

[391] Cole, S.L., et al., *Statins cause intracellular accumulation of amyloid precursor protein, beta-secretase-cleaved fragments, and amyloid beta-peptide via an isoprenoid-dependent mechanism*. J Biol Chem, 2005. 280(19): p. 18755-70.

[392] Ostrowski, S.M., et al., *Statins Reduce Amyloid-beta Production through Inhibition of Protein Isoprenylation*. J Biol Chem, 2007. 282(37): p. 26832-44.

[393] Chauhan, N.B., G.J. Siegel, and D.L. Feinstein, *Effects of lovastatin and pravastatin on amyloid processing and inflammatory response in TgCRND8 brain*. Neurochem Res, 2004. 29(10): p. 1897-911.

[394] Jiang, S., et al., *Trafficking regulation of proteins in Alzheimer's disease*. Mol Neurodegener, 2014. 9: p. 6.

[395] Shinohara, M., et al., *Reduction of brain beta-amyloid (Abeta) by fluvastatin, a hydroxyme-thylglutaryl-CoA reductase inhibitor, through increase in degradation of amyloid precursor protein C-terminal fragments (APP-CTFs) and Abeta clearance*. J Biol Chem, 2010. 285(29): p. 22091-102.

[396] Parsons, R.B. and B.M. Austen, *Protein lipidation of BACE*. Biochem Soc Trans, 2005. 33(Pt 5): p. 1091-3.

[397] Parsons, R.B., et al., *Statins inhibit the dimerization of beta-secretase via both isoprenoid- and cholesterol-mediated mechanisms*. Biochem J, 2006. 399(2): p. 205-14.

[398] Urano, Y., et al., *Association of active gamma-secretase complex with lipid rafts*. J Lipid Res, 2005. 46(5): p. 904-12.

[399] Zhou, Y., et al., *Geranylgeranyl pyrophosphate stimulates gamma-secretase to increase the generation of Abeta and APP-CTFgamma*. FASEB J, 2008. 22(1): p. 47-54.

[400] Kukar, T., et al., *Diverse compounds mimic Alzheimer disease-causing mutations by augmenting Abeta42 production*. Nature medicine, 2005. 11(5): p. 545-50.

[401] Zhou, Y., et al., *Nonsteroidal anti-inflammatory drugs can lower amyloidogenic Abeta42 by inhibiting Rho*. Science, 2003. 302(5648): p. 1215-7.

[402] Selkoe, D.J. and D. Schenk, *Alzheimer's disease: molecular understanding predicts amy-loid-based therapeutics*. Annu Rev Pharmacol Toxicol, 2003. 43: p. 545-84.

[403] Clippingdale, A.B., J.D. Wade, and C.J. Barrow, *The amyloid-beta peptide and its role in Alzheimer's disease*. J Pept Sci, 2001. 7(5): p. 227-49.

[404] Nathalie, P. and O. Jean-Noel, *Processing of amyloid precursor protein and amyloid peptide neurotoxicity.* Curr Alzheimer Res, 2008. 5(2): p. 92-9.

[405] Saido, T.C. and N. Iwata, *Metabolism of amyloid beta peptide and pathogenesis of Alzheimer's disease. Towards presymptomatic diagnosis, prevention and therapy.* Neuroscience research, 2006. 54(4): p. 235-53.

[406] Mawuenyega, K.G., et al., *Decreased clearance of CNS beta-amyloid in Alzheimer's disease.* Science, 2010. 330(6012): p. 1774.

[407] Tamboli, I.Y., et al., *Statins promote the degradation of extracellular amyloid {beta}-peptide by microglia via stimulation of exosome-associated insulin-degrading enzyme (IDE) secretion.* J Biol Chem, 2010. 285(48): p. 37405-14.

[408] Cheng, S., et al., *Farnesyltransferase haplodeficiency reduces neuropathology and rescues cognitive function in a mouse model of Alzheimer disease.* J Biol Chem, 2013. 288(50): p. 35952-60.

[409] Cordle, A. and G. Landreth, *3-Hydroxy-3-methylglutaryl-coenzyme A reductase inhibitors attenuate beta-amyloid-induced microglial inflammatory responses.* The Journal of neuroscience : the official journal of the Society for Neuroscience, 2005. 25(2): p. 299-307.

[410] Cordle, A., et al., *Mechanisms of statin-mediated inhibition of small G-protein function.* The Journal of Biological Chemistry, 2005. 280(40): p. 34202-9.

[411] Kidd, M., *Paired helical filaments in electron microscopy of Alzheimer's disease.* Nature, 1963. 197: p. 192-3.

[412] Iqbal, K., et al., *Tau in Alzheimer disease and related tauopathies.* Curr Alzheimer Res, 2010. 7(8): p. 656-64.

[413] Meske, V., et al., *Blockade of HMG-CoA reductase activity causes changes in microtubule-stabilizing protein tau via suppression of geranylgeranylpyrophosphate formation: implications for Alzheimer's disease.* Eur J Neurosci, 2003. 17(1): p. 93-102.

[414] Hamano, T., et al., *Pitavastatin decreases tau levels via the inactivation of Rho/ROCK.* Neurobiol Aging, 2011.

[415] Barbero-Camps, E., et al., *APP/PS1 mice overexpressing SREBP-2 exhibit combined Abeta accumulation and tau pathology underlying Alzheimer's disease.* Hum Mol Genet, 2013. 22(17): p. 3460-76.

[416] Bolognin, S., et al., *The Potential Role of Rho GTPases in Alzheimer's Disease Pathogenesis.* Mol Neurobiol, 2014.

[417] Huesa, G., et al., *Altered distribution of RhoA in Alzheimer's disease and AbetaPP overexpressing mice.* J Alzheimers Dis, 2010. 19(1): p. 37-56.

[418] Takai, Y., T. Sasaki, and T. Matozaki, *Small GTP-binding proteins.* Physiol Rev, 2001. 81(1): p. 153-208.

[419]   Ng, E.L. and B.L. Tang, *Rab GTPases and their roles in brain neurons and glia*. Brain Res Rev, 2008. 58(1): p. 236-46.

[420]   Ginsberg, S.D., et al., *Regional selectivity of rab5 and rab7 protein upregulation in mild cognitive impairment and Alzheimer's disease*. Journal of Alzheimer's disease : JAD, 2010. 22(2): p. 631-9.

[421]   Ginsberg, S.D., et al., *Upregulation of* select rab GTPases in cholinergic basal forebrain neurons in mild cognitive impairment and Alzheimer's disease. Journal of chemical neuroanatomy, 2011.

[422]   Armstrong, A., et al., Lysosomal Network Proteins as Potential Novel CSF Biomarkers for Alzheimer's Disease. Neuromolecular Med, 2014. 16(1): p. 150-60.

[423]   Scheper, W., et al., Rab6 is increased in Alzheimer's disease brain and correlates with endoplasmic reticulum stress. Neuropathol Appl Neurobiol, 2007. 33(5): p. 523-32.

[424]   Camargo, N., A.B. Smit, and M.H. Verheijen, SREBPs: SREBP function in glia-neuron interactions. FEBS J, 2009. 276(3): p. 628-36.

[425]   Bogdanovic, N., et al., On the turnover of brain cholesterol in patients with Alzheimer's disease. Abnormal induction of the cholesterol-catabolic enzyme CYP46 in glial cells. Neurosci Lett, 2001. 314(1-2): p. 45-8.

7

Metals Involvement in Alzheimer's Disease — A Patho-Genetic View

Carlo Salustri, Mariacristina Siotto,
Serena Bucossi and Rosanna Squitti

Additional information is available at the end of the chapter

1. Introduction

As Alois Alzheimer himself first observed, the brain of an individual affected by Alzheimer's disease (AD) shows aggregations of the peptide beta-amyloid (Aβ) and tau proteins, which form characteristic plaques and neurofibrillary tangles respectively [1].

Since Aβ is known to participate in many normal body functions, its precipitation into plaques, often referred to as 'amyloid cascade', has been for a long time the only recognized, yet unexplained mechanism of AD pathogenesis [2]. In time, however, diverse phenomena, such as oxidative stress, aberrant inflammations, impaired energy metabolism and more have been gradually discovered to contribute to the cascade [3].

The observation that Aβ aggregation in plaques is an age-dependent phenomenon, whereas Aβ production is not, suggested that some other age-dependent mechanism must play a role in transforming Aβ into a neurotoxic element. The fact that some metals, such as copper and zinc, are known to modulate glutamatergic neurotransmission [4] led researchers to hypothesize that late-age abnormalities in the homeostasis of one or more transition metals may play a role in the amyloid cascade.

Moreover, much evidence gathered on AD depicts an improperly functioning ceruloplasmin, an enzyme synthesized by the liver, which controls iron oxidization state. There is also evidence that a functional failure of systemic ceruloplasmin may be behind the iron-related redox processes that produce oxidative stress in the AD brain [5, 6]. Ceruloplasmin is the 'crosstalk' factor linking copper to iron metabolism, thus its failure is very likely to be a major actor in the dysfunctional metal metabolism affecting AD individuals. Aβ may gain toxicity upon some interaction with copper, in a process involving ceruloplasmin, even though the molecular mechanism still remains elusive.

This notion was further supported by the fact that the Amyloid precursor protein (APP) was discovered to possess selective copper binding sites, which mediate redox activities causing precipitation of Aβ even at low concentrations [7]. Aβ itself has been reported to possess selective high- and low-affinity metal-binding sites which, in normal conditions, bind equimolar amounts of either copper or zinc but, in conditions of acidosis, see zinc completely displaced by copper [8]. Thus, hyper-metallation was suggested to be the mechanism that gives Aβ its redox properties, triggering redox cycles through production of H_2O_2 that lead to self-oxidation of Aβ, formation of oligomers with diverse grades of complexity and finally to Aβ precipitation into plaques (Figure 1) [4, 9].

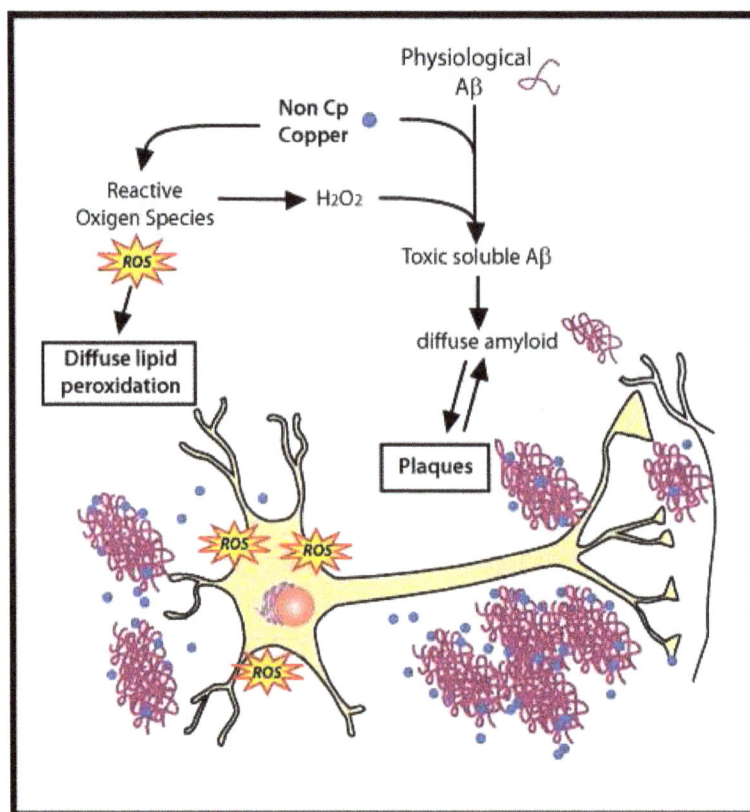

Figure 1. Systemic Non-Cp-copper in AD passes through the Blood Brain Barrier and causes an imbalance of copper in the brain. Here Non-Cp-copper can interact with physiological amyloid-β (Aβ), forming clusters of metal-toxic soluble Aβ that evolve in diffuse amyloid and, finally, in toxic plaques. Non-Cp-Copper can also interact with reactive oxygen species (ROS), which are responsible for lipid peroxidation in neuron membranes, protein oxidation, and cleavage of DNA and RNA molecules.

Diverse animal studies support the toxic role of copper in AD pathogenesis.

White et al. [10] showed that the copper contents of both liver and cerebral cortex in $APP^{-/-}$ and amyloid precursor-like protein $(APLP2^{-/-})$ knockout mice were significantly increased, supporting the authors' hypothesis that the *APP* gene modulates hepatic and cortical copper levels. However, the mechanism leading to increased brain copper content (due to *APP* gene knockout) remains known. Serum copper levels were not significantly more altered in *APP*^{-/-} and *APLP2*^{-/-} mice than in wild-type mice. It appears that a failure of copper excretion from the brain to the blood or, more likely, an imbalance of copper distribution between the Cp-bound and unbound fractions could be associated with the deposition of excessive copper levels in the brain in this knockout model. Besides demonstrating that the AβPP is an important regulator of brain copper homeostasis, White et al. also demonstrated that it potentiates the Aβ-mediated neurotoxicity by increasing oxidative stress.

Sparks and Schreurs [11] demonstrated that adding 0.12 ppm (0.12 mg/L) of copper to water given to a cholesterol-fed rabbit AD-model resulted in significantly enhanced cognitive waning and also exacerbated amyloid plaque deposition. This finding led to serious concerns in some Government Environmental Agencies about the content of copper in drinking water delivered to households via copper pipes. It must be kept in mind that cholesterol, though vital for neuronal transmission, synaptic plasticity and cell function, is also a well-established risk factor for atherosclerosis and AD [12]. Cholesterol to 7-hydroxy cholesterol oxidation, caused by Aβ, is extremely toxic for neurons [13]. Cp levels measured using o-dianisidine dihydrochloride as a substrate in the plasma of cholesterol-fed rabbit model after adding copper to drinking water, suggest an increase, although the change did not reach statistical significance. This suggests that a Non-Cp copper increase is a vehicle of copper within the brain.

In a different investigation [14], Sparks reconfirmed this earlier finding, reporting that other animal models, like spontaneously hyper-cholesterolemic Watanabe rabbits, cholesterol-fed beagles and rabbits, and *PS1* and *APP* transgenic mice showed considerably increased brain levels of Aβ when given copper-rich (0.12 ppm) drinking water. Notably, non-cholesterol fed *PS1* and *APP* transgenic mice models of AD demonstrated significantly enhanced levels of Aβ due to copper exposure via drinking water, demonstrating that the mouse model of AD exhibits vulnerability to copper even in the absence of cholesterol in the diet. This observation highlights the fact that both cholesterol and copper are separate causative factors whose interaction further enhances the formation of Aβ plaques.

In another study [15], Lu at al. confirmed the findings of Sparks and colleagues'. The authors demonstrated that Kunming strain mice fed with a high-cholesterol diet and distilled water containing 0.21 ppm copper exhibited significantly increased level of *APP* mRNA, coupled with the activation of caspase-3 in the brain, suggesting apoptosis mediated neurotoxicity. Strikingly, copper also increased cholesterol-induced learning and memory impairment in mice.

Moreover, it has been reported [16] that, in Sprague-Dawley rats, which underwent bilateral common carotid artery occlusion (2VO) and were administered with 250 ppm copper containing water for 3 months, chronic copper toxicity exacerbated memory impairment induced by 2VO coupled with an augmented expression of brain AβPP and β-site AβPP-cleaving enzyme 1 (BACE1) at both mRNA and protein levels. However, these copper-aggravated changes were ameliorated after copper was withdrawn from the drinking water.

As a whole, these experimental animal models demonstrated the toxicity mediated by copper in the AD cascade, showing that increased level of copper ingested with drinking water, or more generally through the diet, affects AD neuropathology.

All this evidence has eventually led to the proposal of the so called Metal Hypothesis of AD (Bush et al. 2008), which is based on the concept that it is the interaction of Aβ with specific metals, especially copper, that actually drives the amyloid cascade and AD pathogenesis.

One question remained: how does copper actually reach the brain? In fact, we normally ingest copper through the diet - via food, drinking water, beverage, supplements - and copper status in the body is regulated by the balance between duodenal absorption (intestine) and biliary excretion (liver). After crossing the intestinal lumen, copper is transported via portal circulation to the liver, where it is partly stored and partly redistributed to other organs. In the hepatocyte, copper is incorporated into ceruloplasmin, whose dimensions don't allow an easy crossing of the blood-brain-barrier (BBB).

An answer to the question came with the discovery that, although the vast majority of human copper circulates tightly bound to ceruloplasmin [17, 18], a faulty copper metabolism leads to the creation of a small pool of copper that goes into circulation loosely bound to and constantly exchanged among albumin, α2 macroglobulin, peptides, amino acids and other low-molecular-weight compounds. Due to the loose character of the bindings, this portion is normally referred to as Non Ceruloplasmin copper (Non–Cp copper). The key difference between bound (to ceruloplasmin) and Non-Cp copper lies in the fact that the low-molecular-weight compounds can easily cross the BBB [18], thus carrying Non-Cp copper into the brain. There, copper can enter cycles of Haber-Weiss or Fenton reactions producing ·OH, against which our body has no defenses [19], and generate pleiotropic effects on the amyloid cascade [3].

The metal hypothesis has also gained support from consistent reports of enhanced concentrations of labile copper in areas of the brain that are considered critical for AD [20].

There is by now a solid body of literature reporting *in vitro* [8, 21, 22], experimental (reviewed in [23, 24]) and clinical evidence gathered over the last years which have shown that some systemic abnormalities in copper metabolism are shared between the AD and the Wilson's disease (WD). Wilson's disease is the paradigmatic disease of copper toxicosis or accumulation [18]. Although much less severe than in WD, it has been shown that the increases in Non-Cp copper correlate with some typical AD deficits, with the 'core' markers of AD in the cerebrospinal fluid [25], a poor prognosis of the disease [26], and the conversion from Mild Cognitive Impairment (MCI) to full dementia [27]. Meta-analyses have confirmed increased levels of total copper and Non-Cp copper in general circulation of AD patients compared with healthy control subjects [28-30]. A higher intake of copper in the diet was also associated with cognitive decline or with an increase in overall mortality. Specifically, in the 'Chicago Health and Aging Project' (3718 subjects followed from 1993 to 2002), a diet with a content of 2.75 mg / day of copper on average, along with a high saturated and trans fat intake, has been proved to be associated with cognitive decline, which was estimated to be equivalent to an extra nineteen years of aging [31]. In the 'Iowa Women's Health Study' (38772 older women followed from

1986 to 2008), the use of dietary supplements of copper has been shown to be associated with a 18% increase in total mortality [32]. Recently, it was shown that the increase of copper in the soil in 26 provinces and 3 municipal districts in China, between 1991 and 2000, is associated with an increased AD-related mortality. In geographic areas with higher concentrations of copper, the relative risk of AD-related death is 2.6 times higher than that in geographical areas with a lower content copper in the soil [33].

Also results of a recently completed Phase II clinical trial, based on using metal attenuating complexing compounds or Zinc therapy [34-37], appear to support the notion of a copper dysfunction in AD. The available evidence has now reached such a quantitative and qualitative level that the notion of a copper-related phenotype in AD has now started to be accepted [23]. This is a very important step, since many translational hypotheses may develop from this notion, in terms of both diagnostic and prognostic tools, with important repercussions in terms of preventive and therapeutic approaches. However, most of the literature dealing with the relationship between copper and AD focuses on local copper abnormal distribution, especially in those specific areas of the brain that are considered critical for the disease. Recently, this vision has started to appear limited. There is now a bulk of evidence suggesting that all modifications should be viewed in a wider framework of systemic, rather than local, metal dishomeostasis. This concept can be better understood looking at recent studies of the link between the status of serum ceruloplasmin and AD clinical signs and/or Aβ markers in the CSF [23]. Torsdottir et al. [38] reported a decrease in ceruloplasmin activity in AD patients. Lower levels of circulating ceruloplasmin in AD patients with different CSF markers of AD were reported by Brewer's [39], Arnal's [40] and Kessler's [41] groups. In 2008, our laboratory demonstrated a consistent and measurable increase of apo-ceruloplasmin (a defective form of ceruloplasmin, lacking copper and its ferroxidase activity) in the serum and CSF of AD patients [42, 43].

Since both WD and the early-onset form of AD are known to have a genetic origin determining the hereditability of the disease, researchers have embarked in a wide range of studies in the attempt to find genes that cause the late-onset AD or at least contribute to it via damaging phenomena, such as oxidative stress, inflammation, apoptosis or an increased expression of Aβ. In order to encompass as much as possible of the huge genome world, researchers have also embarked in so-called large-scale genome-wide association studies (GWAS). These studies search for DNA sequence variations that appear more common in individuals with a certain disease than in individuals without that disease. GWAS typically analyze a multitude of single gene variations, generally called single-nucleotide polymorphisms (SNPs), and verify their association, if any, with the traits of a disease.

2. AD and *APOE*

So far, no specific gene has been found that can be reliably considered a cause of AD. Even genes, whose mutations have been found responsible for early-onset AD, appear to have a minor, or at least not a pivotal role in the late-onset form. However, numerous risk factors have been identified in the last few years. Historically, the first one to be established is the inheritance of the ε4 allele of the apolipoprotein E (*APOE*), found on chromosome 19. *APOE* is the gene encoding the protein that carries cholesterol and other fats into circulation and manifests itself in a number of alleles, of which ε2, ε3 and ε4 are the most common. The allele ε3, the most common of the three, appears totally unrelated to the risk of developing AD. The slightly less common ε4, instead, has been definitely established to increase the risk of developing AD. The rare variant ε2 seems instead to provide some form of protection by delaying the onset age of the disease.

Individuals inherit two copies of the *APOE* gene, one from each parent, which can be different alleles. If one of the inherited alleles is ε4, the carrier has about a 3-fold increased risk of developing AD. Two copies of ε4 make this risk is much higher, reaching a 15-fold increase of the risk. In other words, it can be stated that *APOE*ε4 carriers have a 90% statistical risk of contracting AD if they are heterozygote and close to 100% if homozygote [44].

It must be emphasized, though, that we are dealing here with statistical risk: in fact, not all individuals who have one or two ε4 develop AD and AD occurs also in people who have no ε4. Thus, *APOE*ε4 is a 'susceptibility' gene, i.e., a gene that affects risk but is not the cause.

3. Other genes

The fact that *APOE*ε4 is neither necessary nor sufficient for the development of the disease has supported the quest for more genetic risk factors and GWAS have led to the identification of numerous genes now widely accepted as risk factors for AD. Major examples include:

CLU – The *CLU* gene on chromosome 8 encodes the protein clusterin, or apolipoprotein J, which is implicated in multiple biological processes, such as lipid transport, membrane recycling, cell adhesion and apoptosis. Two GWAS have independently found a statistical association between a SNP within *CLU* and the risk of having AD [45, 46]. Despite the fact that people who already have AD have more clusterin in their blood, and that clusterin blood levels correlate with faster cognitive decline in individuals with AD, there is no indication that levels of this protein can predict the onset of AD.

SORL1 – an *APOE* receptor in the neural system. Some variants on chromosome 11 have been related to AD [47], since a significant decrease in their expression has been found in AD patients and some authors have described a link between *SORL1* and APP regulation.

CR1 – encodes the protein C3b/C4b receptor, whose deficiency may contribute to chronic inflammation in the brain. Some specific variant of this gene have been identified as contributors to AD [46, 47].

PICALM - located on chromosome 11, encodes phosphatidylinositol-binding clathrin assembly protein, which is linked to the process by which brain nerve cells (neurons) communicate with each other. GWAS have identified several functional SNPs in the *PICALM* gene [45-50]

In AD, GWAS have consistently shown that the effect size and the strength of association of *APOE* variants are greater than the best of *APOE*-unrelated associations. This stresses the relevance of *APOE* as risk factor for AD, although also other explanations should be considered: firstly, most GWAS do not study the variants' true susceptibility but are rather based on the identification of their tagging markers. The latter generally show much greater heterogeneity than the former in terms of both alleles and extent of linkage. Consequently, it is possible that some variants have in reality bigger effect sizes than the ones seen by GWAS. Secondly, current GWAS platforms are often insufficient to detect rare variants. Thus, the existence of some variants that have a big effect size but happen to be rare can remain undetected. Moreover, the linear modeling framework often used in GWASs considers only one SNP at a time, thus ignoring the genomic and environmental context of each SNP [51]. This is an important limitation since the genotype-phenotype relationship is most likely characterized by significant genetic heterogeneity and complex gene-gene and gene-environment interactions [52]. Recently, there has been a shift away from the 'one SNP at a time' method toward a more holistic approach that includes the gene's environmental context.

Another approach is selecting a candidate gene on the basis of hypotheses regarding the disease and then analyze all sequence changes of that gene. Direct sequencing has proven an effective way to discover rare variants with large effect sizes. Recently, studies using next-generation sequencing have led to the identification of rare frequency coding variants in *PLD3* [53] and *TREM2* genes [54, 55] associated with the risk of AD.

3.1. *ATP7A* and *ATP7B*

Two serious disorders are today recognized to be due to a dyshomeostasis in copper metabolism: Menkes disease (MD) and Wilson's disease (WD). Both are caused by a mutation of one gene: *ATP7A* in MD and *ATP7B* in WD, which generate a dysfunction of the proteins they encode: ATP7A and ATP7B, respectively [56]. These two proteins are copper pump proteins or transporting ATPase and, although they have somewhat different distributions in diverse cell types, both are key in regulating copper levels in the body.

The *ATP7A* gene is located on the long (q) arm of the X chromosome. The protein it encodes, ATP7A, is found virtually everywhere in the body except in the liver and delivers copper wherever it is needed within tissue cells. In the small intestine, it contributes to control the absorption of copper from food. Mutations of the *ATP7A* gene lead to synthesis of dysfunctional proteins, of which some engage in disorderly copper transport while others are even unable to bind the metal. More than 100 mutations the have been identified as causes of MD.

ATP7B is a gene of chromosome 13, expressed mainly in the liver, although it has also been detected in the brain, heart, kidney, lung, mammary gland and placenta [57]. The protein it encodes, ATP7B, maintains the body copper homeostasis. In the hepatocyte, ATP7B receives copper from ATOX1 and it moves across the trans Golgi network where it incorporates this metal into apo-ceruloplasmin generating a holo-active form. When intracellular copper levels exceed cell needs, ATP7B moves toward the bile canaliculi and carries out the excretion of copper [58].

Technically, mutations of the two genes have somewhat opposite effects: in MD, the dysfunctional *ATP7A* results in an unbalanced distribution of copper throughout the body. Copper accumulates in some tissues while it remains insufficient in others, where the decreased supply reduces the activity of enzymes that are necessary for the health of numerous body parts, such as bone, skin, blood vessels, and the nervous system. In WD, instead, the dysfunctional ATP7B causes: (i) a failure in the incorporation of copper into the holo-ceruloplasmin, resulting in increased levels of Non-Cp copper being released into the blood stream and in low circulating levels of that protein; (ii) decreased levels of copper released into the bile canaliculi, causing cell over-feeding and intracellular copper deposits, which accelerate apoptotic cell death [59].

We know that in WD huge amounts of Non-Cp copper enter the brain through the BBB, where labile copper accumulates and leads to neurodegeneration. WD is considered the hallmark of copper toxicosis.

Since increased copper levels characterizing WD are shared in a smaller scale by AD patients, the *ATP7B* gene and its variations have of course become the focus of much of our research focusing on copper. Some authors have expressed doubts about this research direction by pointing out that neurodegeneration in WD leads to movement disorders with little or no effect on cognition, while AD neurodegeneration affects chiefly cognition. Moreover, onset ages are very different in the two pathologies as WD appears typically in childhood, whereas late-onset AD by definition after 60-65y. In other words, even accepting the fact that the two pathologies share copper toxicity, manifestations are so different that it seems unreasonable to claim that the same gene causes both of them. In reply to this valid concern, other authors have argued that *ATP7B* has a high variability. Thus, the possibility that this gene is a causative gene for WD when in homozygosis and a susceptibility gene for AD (interacting with environmental factors and other risk genes) cannot be ruled out. Other genes have shown unexpected diverse effects. *ATP7A*, for example, which is causative of MD, has been recently recognized to be associated with a mild form of occipital horn syndrome [60]. Moreover, recent evidence has demonstrated that certain missense mutations of this gene can cause a syndrome restricted to progressive distal motor neuropathy even without signs of copper deficiency [61].

Our laboratory has pursued the link between copper and AD pathogenesis on the assumption that the excessive Non-Cp copper production in the body is actually due to a faulty ATP7B causing a flaw in the incorporation of copper into nascent ceruloplasmin in the liver [56]. On this basis, we have embarked in an extensive study of the *ATP7B* gene and of the protein ATP7B, which is the only one known to catalyze that incorporation.

Unfortunately, analysis of the *ATP7B* gene is not an easy task, due to its huge variability. The 1000 Genomes project has identified 1,358 variations of *ATP7B* in human populations. At least 500 of them have been recognized as disease-causing [62]. Worldwide detection of *ATP7B* mutations is actually difficult [63] since most mutations are rare, reported only within single families and often prevalent in specific ethnic groups [32]. As a result, the database regarding both the gene's properties and the possible dysfunctions of the proteins they encode is still largely insufficient [64].

The first significant information on the structure of the ATP7B protein was gained from a homology modeling study [65]. Some more light was later shed by nuclear magnetic resonance (NMR) spectroscopy studies [66-70]. Recently, significant progress in the comprehension of

ATP7B structural organization has come from the solution of the crystal structure of the bacterial copper ATPase LCopA [71]. The LCopA protein model has been employed as a template to analyze ATP7B core domain on the basis of its sequence homology to build interpretations of WD mutations [64].

We know that mutations leading to a complete abolition of ATP7B function, chiefly early stop mutations and mutations in regions of the gene that have a high functional importance, lead to an early and predominantly hepatic dysfunction. Conversely, point mutations in regions that are functionally less important are associated with a later onset and predominantly neurological or psychiatric dysfunctions [17].

An effective strategy to characterize genetic compositions, which has become popular in recent years, is the so-called *in-silico* analysis, i.e., performed via computer simulations. Several computational procedures have been developed to analyze the effects of genetic variants on the protein function. The advantage of this type of analysis is that it allows analysis of huge amounts of data, delivered by high-throughput sequencing technologies, in relatively short time. These procedures take into account different factors associated with the protein properties, such as chemistry constraints, three dimensional structure, and amino acid sequences of homologous and orthologous proteins [72].

Our laboratory has used a new in-silico approach based on amino acid sequence, utilizing four among the most used bioinformatics tools (i.e. Polyphen- 2, SIFT, Panther, and PhD-SNPs). We have applied this approach to non-synonymous SNP (nsSNPs) detected in the *ATP7B* gene to profile WD-causing and WD-non-causing mutations, while obtaining at the same time useful information about the gene's domains that could potentially harbor loci of susceptibility for other disorders related to copper metabolism [73].

3.2. rs7323774 and rs2147363

In pursuit of the identification of regions in the *ATP7B* gene linked to copper dishomeostasis, our laboratory has embarked in an investigation of the association between copper-related biochemical markers in serum (bound copper, Non-Cp copper and ceruloplasmin) and variants of the *ATP7B* gene.

In one study of 399 AD patients and 303 healthy elderly controls, we focused our attention on a set of four SNPs that had been reported to be informative of the *ATP7B* gene structure [74]: rs1801243 (missense substitution: Ser406Ala), rs2147363 (intronic variant: c.1544-53A>C), rs1061472 (missense substitution: Lys832Arg) and rs732774 (missense substitution: Arg952Lys). We had already found in a previous study that those SNPs among the four that lay in the transmembrane domains appear to have an association with AD [75].

We first stratified the AD and control groups into three 'classes' according to their Non-Cp copper levels: 'low Non-Cp copper' (<1 μmol/L), 'medium Non-Cp copper' (≥1, <1.6 μmol/L) and 'high Non-Cp copper' (≥1.6 μmol/L) (Figure 2). Results showed antithetic distributions for patients and controls: the 'low Non-Cp copper' class accounted for 27% of AD cases vs. 61% of controls; the 'medium Non-Cp copper' for 11% of AD vs. 10% of controls and the 'high Non-Cp copper' for 62% of AD versus 29% of controls. The serum copper profile was then analyzed in relation to the selected gene variants in the sole 'high Non-Cp copper' class (patients with AD, n = 109; controls, n = 53).

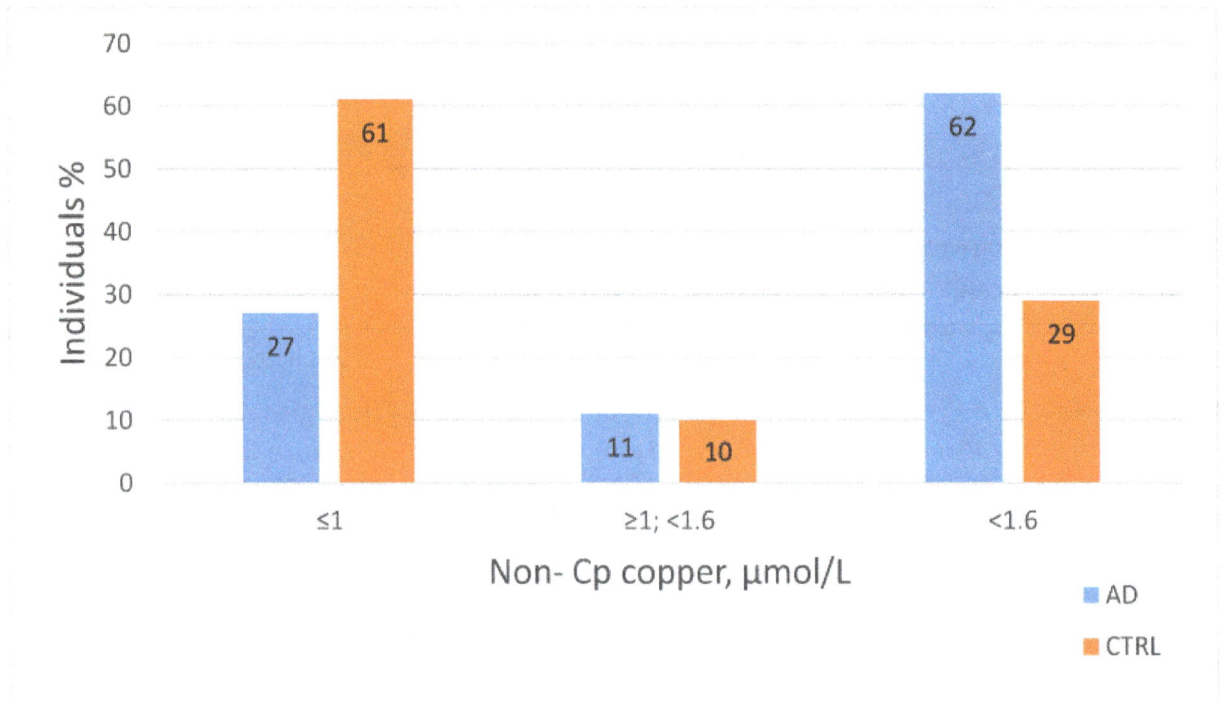

Figure 2. Stratification of the AD and control groups (CTRL) into three 'classes' according to their Non-Cp copper levels: 'low Non-Cp copper' (<1 µmol/L), 'medium Non-Cp copper' (≥1, <1.6 µmol/L) and 'high Non-Cp copper' (≥1.6 µmol/L). The bar graph reports the percentage of AD (first bar from left) and CTRL (second bar from left) for each class.

The main result of this study was that individuals who are GG homozygous for *ATP7B* rs7323774 SNP have higher levels of Non-Cp copper in their serum. This was true for the entire sample of patients and controls but was definitely more pronounced in AD individuals. Non-Cp copper distributions of AD patients turned out antithetic to those of controls and results showed that this is due to those *ATP7B* variants that are located in regions encoding ATP7B transmembrane domains, i.e., variants that we know to be associated with copper dyshomeostasis in AD. It must be noted, however, that we selected the variants on the basis of the information they could deliver on the *ATP7B* gene structure, not for their impact on gene function. Consequently, it is obvious that rs1801243, rs2147363, rs1061472 and rs732774, even though significantly associated with AD [74], could not be the loci responsible for the effects of the *ATP7B* gene on AD, either in terms of Non-Cp copper derangement or in terms of an increased risk of the AD [76].

In another study of 286 AD patients and 283 controls we focused on the rs2147363 and rs7334118 variants of the *ATP7B* gene. All genotype frequencies in our controls were within the ranges reported previously in the European origin populations of the HapMap project (available on http://hapmap.ncbi.nlm.nih.gov).

We analyzed the genetic association between SNPs and AD risk. Our study revealed a significant association between rs2147363 and AD. When data were adjusted for confounding variables (i.e., age, gender, and *APOE* genotype), significant results were obtained for the recessive model (OR: 1.63, 95% CI: 1.03–2.57; p = 0.035) and Log-additive model (OR: 1.51, 95% CI: 1.05–2.16; p = 0.025).

In order to verify whether rs2147363 has any functional variants in LD, we also analyzed the SNPs that showed a complete LD (D' = 1) with this *ATP7B* variant in Tuscans in Italy (TSI), which is the HapMap population most genetically related to our sample. We identified ten SNPs in complete LD with the rs2147363. We prioritized these variants using FastSNP. This analysis highlighted that one variant is a non-synonymous SNP (medium-high risk), four are intronic enhancers (very low-low risk), four are intronic with no known function (no effect), and one is a downstream variant with no known function (no effect) (Table 1).

SNP ID (rs)	Possible Functional Effects	Region	SIFT	PolyPhen2
rs7334118	*Missense (non-conservative); Splicing regulation*	*coding*	*Damaging*	*Possibly Damaging*
rs4943053	Intronic enhancer	intronic	-	-
rs9535803	Intronic enhancer	intronic	-	-
rs9535809	Intronic enhancer	intronic	-	-
rs2147362	Intronic enhancer	intronic	-	-
rs11839458	Intronic with unknown function	intronic	-	-
rs9526820	Intronic with unknown function	intronic	-	-
rs9535827	Intronic with unknown function	intronic	-	-
rs9535794	Downstream with unknown function	3-UTR	-	-
rs9535806	Intronic with unknown function	intronic	-	-

Table 1. Prioritization and functional analysis of *ATP7B* SNPs in LD with **rs2147363**.

To predict the functional impact of the non-synonymous SNP (rs7334118), we used two different bioinformatics tools: SIFT and Polyphen2. The application of both the SIFT algorithm using orthologous sequences and the Polyphen2 tool highlighted that this coding variant may have an adverse effect on the ATP7B protein.

To verify the hypothesis that genetic association of rs2147363 is due to LD with the rs7334118 SNP, 176 AD subjects and 169 healthy controls among the study population were genotyped for the SNP rs7334118. Two AD patients were carriers of the rs7334118G allele, whereas no healthy individual with this *ATP7B* mutation was identified. Even though this coding variant was identified only in AD patients, its allele frequency in the AD group is in line with the minor allele frequency observed in a general population of European origin (information available at dbSNP). Thus, this result has to be confirmed in a bigger healthy control sample.

To test whether the intronic region, in which rs2147363 is located, plays a role in the regulation of the *ATP7B* gene function, the GERP++ and is-rSNP algorithms were used. rs2147363 nucleotide position resulted non-conserved, whereas, in the intronic region around this SNP, 7 nucleotide positions on the 16 analyzed (43%) achieve the GERP threshold [77]. Table 2 describes the findings of the is-rSNP algorithm. This analysis predicted the presence of binding sites of 8 transcription factors (TF) binding sites, and, in two cases (i.e., Zfp423 and PLAG1), the prediction results were significant (adjusted $p < 0.05$). The main result of this detailed genetic analysis is that the significant association between rs2147363 SNP and AD can be explained on the basis of the presence of TFs binding sites in the region in which this variant is located. Thereby, rs2147363 may be associated with a cis-regulatory function. Specifically, we observed two of the genetic models of rs2147363 SNP associated with AD: a recessive model that suggested a 1.63-fold increased, and a log-additive model that suggested a 1.51-fold increase in the risk of having AD. The Akaike Information Criterion (AIC) and Bayesian Information Criterion (BIC) analyses highlighted that log-additive model achieved the most reliable outcome. This suggests that C allele of rs2147363 SNP is additive: its presence in one gene copy will lead to an increase in AD risk; its presence in both gene copies will lead to a further increase. Additionally, we tested the reliability of our coding or noncoding hypotheses to explain this intronic association. When we considered the coding hypothesis, we analyzed the SNPs in complete LD (D' = 1) with rs2147363 in TSI. The functional prediction analysis showed that the SNP rs7334118 has a complete LD (D' = 1) with rs2147363. Moreover, rs7334118 has been recorded in the Wilson's Disease Mutation database (available at http://www.wilson-disease.med. ualberta.ca) and in Human Genome Mutation Database (available at http:// www.hgmd.cf.ac.uk/) as a Wilson's disease-causing variant, it corresponds to H1207R, located into the P-domain, the domain in which phosphorylation of ATP7B occurs; in particular the residue lies in the ATP-hinge which connects the nucleotide-binding domain (N-domain) and the P-domain (Figure 3). Even though the genotype analysis in our case-control population revealed the presence of two carriers of the rs7334118G allele in AD patients and none in healthy controls, this *ATP7B* mutation could not alone explain the genetic association observed for rs2147363. Specifically, two AD patients heterozygous for the rs7334118G mutation were also carriers of the C allele in rs2147363 (1%). On the contrary, the other 166 AD patients, carriers of the C allele in rs2147363, were negative for the rs7334118 WD mutation (99%). However, this result does not exclude additional rare variants with large functional effects may explain this intronic association.

We used the HapMap database to identify functional coding variants, in which only few rare variants are present. Using other genomic databases, such as the database of 1,000 Genomes Project, may deliver new candidate variants that could be tested to explain our intronic association. Conversely, in-silico analyses on rs2147363 revealed that this intronic SNP can have a regulatory role on ATP7B function. In particular, the GERP analysis highlighted that the intronic region around rs2147363 resulted significantly conserved, and the is-rSNP algorithm significantly predicted the presence of two TF-binding sites in the rs2147363 region. These independent findings suggested that this genomic region has a regulatory function, and consequently rs2147363 can be associated with clinical phenotypes related to ATP7B dysfunction.

Position	Nucleotide	GERP++ score
chr13: 52542783	**C**	**2.17**
chr13: 52542784	**A**	**2.37**
chr13: 52542785	G	-7.84
chr13: 52542786	**G**	**4.09**
chr13: 52542787	G	0.889
chr13: 52542788	C	-1.02
chr13: 52542789	C	1.93
chr13: 52542790	T	-0.596
chr13: 52542791	**C**	**4.11**
chr13: 52542792	T	-3.02
chr13: 52542793	**A**	**2.98**
chr13: 52542794	G	-3.44
chr13: 52542795	**G**	**2.55**
chr13: 52542796	T	-7.19
chr13: 52542797	**T**	**3.25**
chr13: 52542798	**G**	**4.87**

Table 2. GERP analysis of the genomic region around rs2147363. Conserved positions are highlighted in bold.

Specifically, Zfp423 and PLAG1 have been predicted to have a binding-site in the genetic region of rs2147363. Both these TFs are involved in complex metabolic processes. For example, Zfp423 has been reported to regulate neural and adipocyte development [78], whereas *PLAG1* is a proto-oncogene that activates genes involved in uncontrolled cell proliferation (e.g., *IGFII*, *CRLF1*, *CRABP2*, *CRIP2*, and *PIGF*) [79]. In this framework, our data on Zfp423 support the hypothesis that *ATP7B* can be involved in molecular pathways linked to brain activity regulation, suggesting new perspectives in the interpretation of neurologic signs of WD and AD. This conclusion fits well with our original hypothesis that *ATP7B* can harbor variants that may account for some of the missing hereditability of AD [80]. In particular, the present data furnished a new insight into the copper hypothesis: non-coding regions can play a role in the *ATP7B* function, and, thereby, genetic variation in *ATP7B* cis-regulatory elements within non-coding regions may be associated with AD risk. Furthermore, genetic data adjusted for age confounding effect confirmed the association between rs2147363 and AD risk. However, although in-silico analyses support our hypothesis, further functional studies are necessary to confirm the role of non-coding variants in the *ATP7B* gene function and in AD risk.

SNPs	Exon	ATP7B sequence NM_000053.3:c	ATP7B sequence NP_000044.2:p	ATP7B domains
rs1801243	2	1216T>G	missense substitution: Ser406Ala	Metal Binding Unit 4
rs2147363	Intron 3	1544-53A>C	-	-
rs1061472	10	2495A>G	missense substitution: Lys832Arg	A-domain
rs732774	12	2855G>A	missense substitution: Arg952Lys	Luminal Loop between TM5-TM6
Linkage Disequilibrium				
rs7334118	17	3620A>G	missense substitution: His1207Arg	P-domain: ATP hinge

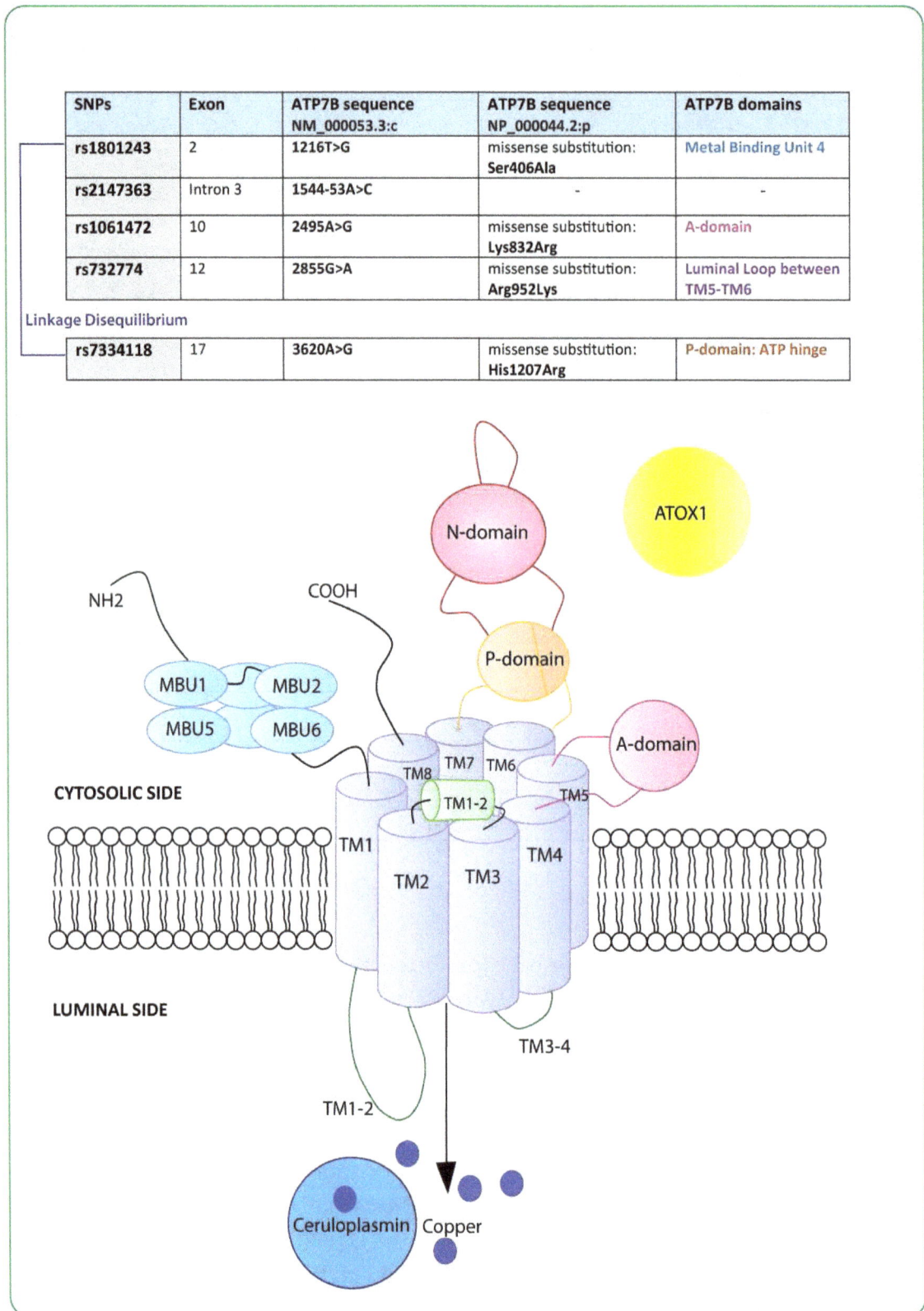

Figure 3. Schematic representation of human ATP7B on the basis of homology-modeled structure [71]. The table reports the *ATP7B* SNPs studied from our group and the specific nucleotide and amino acid substitutions, standing in a specific ATP7B domain.

3.3. K832R (rs1061472) and R952K (rs732774)

In a recent study, we focused our attention on two functional changes in the *ATP7B* gene in particular: K832R (rs1061472) and R952K (rs732774).

K832R corresponds to a non synonymous amino acid substitution and the corresponding AAG>AGG mutation in exon 10 specifies this amino acid change in the A-domain, within the ATP binding domain region of the protein. R952K (AGA>AAA) corresponds to a non-synonymous substitution in the loop between Tm 5-Tm6 of the protein (Figure 3). Our aim was to verify whether and in what way these amino acid changes have a disturbing effect on the function of the ATP7B protein in terms of metal binding properties or ATP hydrolysis, which can eventually result in copper dyshomeostasis.

We recruited 251 AD patients and 201 controls. As reported in the original article [76], for the K832R substitution, the minor allele frequency (MAF) resulted 40% in Italian Tuscans, 45% in Utah residents with Northern and Western European ancestry, while 42% in our controls. For the R952K substitution, MAF was 39% in Italian Tuscans, 44% in Utah residents and 43% in controls. The LD analysis revealed an association between K832R and R952K substitutions in both AD patients (D′ = 0.79) and controls (D′ = 0.81). A high LD between K832R and R952K was confirmed also in all HapMap populations.

Allele frequency distributions of both *ATP7B* SNPs differed between AD and controls: K832R substitution genotype frequencies were K832/K832 10%, K832/R832 47%, and R832/R832 43% ($\chi 2$ test, p = 0.022) in AD patients, while K832/K832 15%, K832/R832 54%, and R832/R832 31% in our controls. R832/R832 genotype was more frequent in AD and this frequency variation was maintained also when taking into account the Bonferroni correction (α= 0.025) as well as in the logistic regression analysis, which took into account age and gender as confounding factors. Our analysis revealed that patients with the *ATP7B* homozygous R832 genotype had a 1.71-fold higher risk of developing AD than controls [adjusted OR= 1.71 (1.12–2.60); p = 0.012]. Genotype frequencies of the R952K substitution were R952/R952 15%, R952/K952 41%, and K952/K952 45% in AD patients, and R952/R952 16%, R952/K952 54%, and K952/K952 30% in our controls.

The $\chi 2$ test indicated that two distributions differed (p = 0.006) and the association between the risk allele K952 and AD was maintained after checking for age and gender as possible confounders in a logistic regression model. In summary, patients with the *ATP7B* homozygous K952 genotype had a 1.82-fold increased risk of AD compared with controls [adjusted OR= 1.82 (1.19–2.80); p = 0.006].

We also performed a haplotype association analysis for the two SNPs in order to investigate their combined effect on AD risk. The most common haplotype was R832/K952, which contained a risk allele at each SNP locus. It was distributed as follows: 60.2% in AD patients and 53.2% in controls (X2 = 4.85; p = 0.028).

The second more frequent haplotype was K832/R952, which contained no risk alleles and its frequencies differed between the two cohorts, being 28.8% in patients and 37.3% in controls (X2 = 7.21; p = 0.007).

A logistic regression model was used to check these associations when taking into account age as a possible confounder. The model confirmed the association (p = 0.018) and revealed that the haplotype K832/R952 confers some protection against AD [adjusted OR= 0.68 (0.49–0.93)]. Thus, the haplotype association analysis revealed that the presence of alleles with normal function, i.e., K832 and R952, is protective, even though the haplotype lies in a gene with significant disease-risk.

It is important to notice that the SNPs of *APOEε4* and *ATP7B* (both K832R and R952K) are independent AD risk factors, as there was no difference in the frequency of the *ATP7B* alleles between carriers and non-carriers of the *APOEε4* variant (consistently p > 0.2), even when the analysis was restricted to assessment of only the AD population (consistently p > 0.2). In summary, the RR genotype in K832R raises the relative risk of developing AD by 71%, while KK in R952K by 82%. The haplotype R832/K952, instead, appears to confer protection against the disease by reducing the relative risk by 32%. These results seem in conflict with the fact that GWASs carried out so far have never found an association between AD and the 13q14.3 chromosomal region where the *ATP7B* gene lies. However, we already described above how GWAS, which are not well equipped to detect rare variants and fail to take into account the genomic and environmental context of the investigated diseases, may underestimate *ATP7B* haplotypes that are instead significantly associated with high risk of AD in individuals exposed to inorganic copper [80].

4. Conclusions

The form of AD that has been the subject of this chapter accounts for about 95% of all AD cases and appears rather late in life, normally after 60. For this reason it is called late-onset Alzheimer's disease (LOAD), a term that well differentiates it from the inherited form, familial AD, which is called early-onset AD because it develops much before 60 and accounts for the remainder 5%. In opposition to familial AD, LOAD was initially called "sporadic" because early researchers saw no link between the disease and hereditary factors and assumed that the appearance of the disease was occasional and totally casual.

As we have seen above, this appeared untrue later, when researchers discovered the role of several polymorphisms of the *APOE* gene in the disease pathogenesis. The term sporadic continued to be widely used but we now know that LOAD is strongly influenced by both genetic and environmental factors and appears to have a complex pattern of inheritance. It remains true, however, that so far no gene has been found to be fully causative of LOAD, a fact that is often referred to as *missing heritability*.

Due to the lack of a secure culprit, the role of genetic mutations in LOAD is often understated. In an attempt to compensate, this chapter has described some of the most meaningful evidence constituting the genetic background believed to provide a combined contribution to susceptibility (to become sick), which remains a statistical entity. It must be kept in mind that not only genetic heterogeneity contributes to susceptibility but also other factors, such as *reduced penetration*, a term describing that a predisposing genotype might be present without the pathology necessarily appearing, or even *phenocopy*, in which there are no predisposing genotypes and yet the pathology develops due to environmental factors. The distinction between *genetic inheritance* and *genetic risk* is fundamental and has helped understand how the disease incidence can be decreased by changes in life style.

The chapter has also described GWAS, which have linked a substantial number of genes to the pathogenesis of AD. It is important to notice that each gene, when taken alone, accounts only for a small percentage of the disease incidence and often lacks clinical significance: the above mentioned *CLU* gene, for example, has a proven correlation with AD-related cognitive decline but its odds ratio tells us that it increases the risk of developing LOAD just 0.1-0.15 times. Moreover, this gene has no clinical relevance since it does not predict the disease onset.

However, all the genetic evidence presented here should be regarded as the framework in which systemic metal unbalances develop. For this reason, we have described in a consequential but also factual fashion the role of systemic copper in the toxic processes leading to AD, which we believe to be among the most important phenomena in AD pathogenesis.

We conclude with the introduction of an important, and somewhat innovative, notion concerning copper in AD. We have shown how multiple variants of the *APOE* gene have an actual effect on the statistical risk to develop AD and how they are also linked to level variations of the portion of copper that does not bind to ceruloplasmin. These variants are also in linkage disequilibrium with rare mutations, which can have a relevant effect on the risk of the disease. We are now starting to explore this field by searching for multiple rare variants in the *ATP7B* gene, which may account for portions of the odds of developing AD, defining a new gene for AD susceptibility. Looking at all these associations as a whole, genetics appears as the factor guiding the association between copper abnormalities and the clinical picture of the disease. In other words, the fact that *ATP7B* multiple rare variants in practice modify the copper homeostasis of an individual and have an effect on his/her risk of developing AD is an expression of the causative character of this gene on the susceptibility of the disease.

Author details

Carlo Salustri[1], Mariacristina Siotto[2], Serena Bucossi[3] and Rosanna Squitti[3,4]

1 Institute of Cognitive Sciences and Technologies (CNR), Fatebenefratelli Hospital, Isola Tiberina, Rome, Italy

2 Don Carlo Gnocchi Foundation ONLUS, Milan, Italy

3 Laboratory of Neurodegeneration, IRCCS San Raffaele Pisana, Rome, Italy

4 Fatebenefratelli Foundation, AFaR Division; Fatebenefratelli Hospital, Isola Tiberina, Rome, Italy

References

[1] Querfurth, H.W. and F.M. LaFerla. *Alzheimer's disease.* N Engl J Med 2010;362(4) 329-44.

[2] Hardy, J.A. and G.A. Higgins. *Alzheimer's disease: the amyloid cascade hypothesis.* Science 1992;256(5054) 184-5.

[3] Frautschy, S.A. and G.M. Cole. *Why pleiotropic interventions are needed for Alzheimer's disease.* Mol Neurobiol 2010;41(2-3) 392-409.

[4] Bush, A.I. and R.E. Tanzi. *Therapeutics for Alzheimer's disease based on the metal hypothesis.* Neurotherapeutics 2008;5(3) 421-32.

[5] Loeffler, D.A., et al. *Increased regional brain concentrations of ceruloplasmin in neurodegenerative disorders.* Brain Res 1996;738(2) 265-74.

[6] Squitti, R., et al. *Ceruloplasmin/Transferrin ratio changes in Alzheimer's disease.* Int J Alzheimers Dis 2010;2011 231595.

[7] Multhaup, G., et al. *The amyloid precursor protein of Alzheimer's disease in the reduction of copper(II) to copper(I).* Science 1996;271(5254) 1406-9.

[8] Atwood, C.S., et al. *Copper catalyzed oxidation of Alzheimer Abeta.* Cell Mol Biol (Noisy-le-grand) 2000;46(4) 777-83.

[9] Cherny, R.A., et al. *Aqueous dissolution of Alzheimer's disease Abeta amyloid deposits by biometal depletion.* J Biol Chem 1999;274(33) 23223-8.

[10] White, A.R., et al. *Copper levels are increased in the cerebral cortex and liver of APP and APLP2 knockout mice.* Brain Res 1999;842(2) 439-44.

[11] Sparks, D.L. and B.G. Schreurs. *Trace amounts of copper in water induce beta-amyloid plaques and learning deficits in a rabbit model of Alzheimer's disease.* Proc Natl Acad Sci U S A 2003;100(19) 11065-9.

[12] Atwood, C.S., et al. *Dramatic aggregation of Alzheimer abeta by Cu(II) is induced by conditions representing physiological acidosis.* J Biol Chem 1998;273(21) 12817-26.

[13] Nelson, T.J. and D.L. Alkon. *Oxidation of cholesterol by amyloid precursor protein and beta-amyloid peptide.* J Biol Chem 2005;280(8) 7377-87.

[14] Sparks, D.L., et al. *Trace copper levels in the drinking water, but not zinc or aluminum influence CNS Alzheimer-like pathology.* J Nutr Health Aging 2006;10(4) 247-54.

[15] Lu, J., et al. *Trace amounts of copper induce neurotoxicity in the cholesterol-fed mice through apoptosis.* FEBS Lett 2006;580(28-29) 6730-40.

[16] Mao, X., et al. *The effects of chronic copper exposure on the amyloid protein metabolisim associated genes' expression in chronic cerebral hypoperfused rats.* Neurosci Lett 2012;518(1) 14-8.

[17] Hoogenraad, T., *Wilson's disease.* 2001, Amsterdam/Rotterdam: Intermed Medical Publishers

[18] Scheinberg, I.H. and I. Sternlieb. *Wilson's Disease.* Annu Rev Med 1965;16 119-34.

[19] Gutteridge, J.M. and B. Halliwell. *The measurement and mechanism of lipid peroxidation in biological systems.* Trends Biochem Sci 1990;15(4) 129-35.

[20] James, S.A., et al. *Elevated labile Cu is associated with oxidative pathology in Alzheimer disease.* Free Radic Biol Med 2012;52(2) 298-302.

[21] Atwood, C.S., et al. *Copper mediates dityrosine cross-linking of Alzheimer's amyloid-beta.* Biochemistry 2004;43(2) 560-8.

[22] White, A.R., et al. *The Alzheimer's disease amyloid precursor protein modulates copper-induced toxicity and oxidative stress in primary neuronal cultures.* J Neurosci 1999;19(21) 9170-9.

[23] Pal, A., et al. *Towards a Unified Vision of Copper Involvement in Alzheimer's Disease: A Review Connecting Basic, Experimental, and Clinical Research.* J Alzheimers Dis 2014.

[24] Squitti, R., M. Siotto, and R. Polimanti. *Low-copper diet as a preventive strategy for Alzheimer's disease.* Neurobiol Aging 2014;35 Suppl 2 S40-50.

[25] Squitti, R., et al. *Excess of nonceruloplasmin serum copper in AD correlates with MMSE, CSF [beta]-amyloid, and h-tau.* Neurology 2006;67(1) 76-82.

[26] Squitti, R., et al. *Longitudinal prognostic value of serum "free" copper in patients with Alzheimer disease.* Neurology 2009;72(1) 50-5.

[27] Squitti, R., et al. *Value of serum nonceruloplasmin copper for prediction of mild cognitive impairment conversion to Alzheimer disease.* Ann Neurol 2014;75(4) 574-80.

[28] Bucossi, S., et al. *Copper in Alzheimer's disease: a meta-analysis of serum,plasma, and cerebrospinal fluid studies.* J Alzheimers Dis 2011;24(1) 175-85.

[29] Schrag, M., et al. *Oxidative stress in blood in Alzheimer's disease and mild cognitive impairment: a meta-analysis.* Neurobiol Dis 2013;59 100-10.

[30] Squitti, R., et al. *Meta-analysis of serum non-ceruloplasmin copper in Alzheimer's disease.* J Alzheimers Dis 2014;38(4) 809-22.

[31] Morris, M.C., et al. *Dietary copper and high saturated and trans fat intakes associated with cognitive decline.* Arch Neurol 2006;63(8) 1085-8.

[32] Mursu, J., et al. *Dietary supplements and mortality rate in older women: the Iowa Women's Health Study.* Arch Intern Med 2011;171(18) 1625-33.

[33]   Shen, X.L., et al. *Positive Relationship between Mortality from Alzheimer's Disease and Soil Metal Concentration in Mainland China.* J Alzheimers Dis 2014;42(3) 893-900.

[34]   Brewer, G.J. *Copper excess, zinc deficiency, and cognition loss in Alzheimer's disease.* Biofactors 2012;38(2) 107-13.

[35]   Lannfelt, L., et al. *Safety, efficacy, and biomarker findings of PBT2 in targeting Abeta as a modifying therapy for Alzheimer's disease: a phase IIa, double-blind, randomised, placebo-controlled trial.* Lancet Neurol 2008;7(9) 779-86.

[36]   Ritchie, C.W., et al. *Metal-protein attenuation with iodochlorhydroxyquin (clioquinol) targeting Abeta amyloid deposition and toxicity in Alzheimer disease: a pilot phase 2 clinical trial.* Arch Neurol 2003;60(12) 1685-91.

[37]   Squitti, R., et al. *d-penicillamine reduces serum oxidative stress in Alzheimer's disease patients.* Eur J Clin Invest 2002;32(1) 51-9.

[38]   Torsdottir, G., et al. *Ceruloplasmin and iron proteins in the serum of patients with Alzheimer's disease.* Dement Geriatr Cogn Dis Extra 2011;1(1) 366-71.

[39]   Brewer, G.J., et al. *Copper and ceruloplasmin abnormalities in Alzheimer's disease.* Am J Alzheimers Dis Other Demen 2010;25(6) 490-7.

[40]   Arnal, N., et al. *Clinical utility of copper, ceruloplasmin, and metallothionein plasma determinations in human neurodegenerative patients and their first-degree relatives.* Brain Res 2010;1319 118-30.

[41]   Kessler, H., et al. *Cerebrospinal fluid diagnostic markers correlate with lower plasma copper and ceruloplasmin in patients with Alzheimer's disease.* J Neural Transm 2006;113(11) 1763-9.

[42]   Capo, C.R., et al. *Features of ceruloplasmin in the cerebrospinal fluid of Alzheimer's disease patients.* Biometals 2008;21(3) 367-72.

[43]   Squitti, R., et al. *Ceruloplasmin fragmentation is implicated in 'free' copper deregulation of Alzheimer's disease.* Prion 2008;2(1) 23-7.

[44]   Corder, E.H., et al. *Gene dose of apolipoprotein E type 4 allele and the risk of Alzheimer's disease in late onset families.* Science 1993;261(5123) 921-3.

[45]   Harold, D., et al. *Genome-wide association study identifies variants at CLU and PICALM associated with Alzheimer's disease.* Nat Genet 2009;41(10) 1088-93.

[46]   Lambert, J.C., et al. *Genome-wide association study identifies variants at CLU and CR1 associated with Alzheimer's disease.* Nat Genet 2009;41(10) 1094-9.

[47]   Lambert, J.C., et al. *Meta-analysis of 74,046 individuals identifies 11 new susceptibility loci for Alzheimer's disease.* Nat Genet 2013;45(12) 1452-8.

[48]   Naj, A.C., et al. *Common variants at MS4A4/MS4A6E, CD2AP, CD33 and EPHA1 are associated with late-onset Alzheimer's disease.* Nat Genet 2011;43(5) 436-41.

[49]   Seshadri, S., et al. *Genome-wide analysis of genetic loci associated with Alzheimer disease.* JAMA 2010;303(18) 1832-40.

[50]   Corneveaux, J.J., et al. *Association of CR1, CLU and PICALM with Alzheimer's disease in a cohort of clinically characterized and neuropathologically verified individuals.* Hum Mol Genet 2010;19(16) 3295-301.

[51]   Moore, J.H., F.W. Asselbergs, and S.M. Williams. *Bioinformatics challenges for genome-wide association studies.* Bioinformatics 2010;26(4) 445-55.

[52]   Stranger, B.E., E.A. Stahl, and T. Raj. *Progress and promise of genome-wide association studies for human complex trait genetics.* Genetics 2011;187(2) 367-83.

[53]   Cruchaga, C., et al. *Rare coding variants in the phospholipase D3 gene confer risk for Alzheimer's disease.* Nature 2014;505(7484) 550-4.

[54]   Guerreiro, R., et al. *TREM2 variants in Alzheimer's disease.* N Engl J Med 2013;368(2) 117-27.

[55]   Jonsson, T., et al. *Variant of TREM2 associated with the risk of Alzheimer's disease.* N Engl J Med 2013;368(2) 107-16.

[56]   Gaggelli, E., et al. *Copper homeostasis and neurodegenerative disorders (Alzheimer's, prion, and Parkinson's diseases and amyotrophic lateral sclerosis).* Chem Rev 2006;106(6) 1995-2044.

[57]   Michalczyk, A.A., et al. *Defective localization of the Wilson disease protein (ATP7B) in the mammary gland of the toxic milk mouse and the effects of copper supplementation.* Biochem J 2000;352 Pt 2 565-71.

[58]   Lutsenko, S., et al. *Function and regulation of human copper-transporting ATPases.* Physiol Rev 2007;87(3) 1011-46.

[59]   Behari, M. and V. Pardasani. *Genetics of Wilsons disease.* Parkinsonism Relat Disord 2010;16(10) 639-44.

[60]   Moller, L.B., et al. *Similar splice-site mutations of the ATP7A gene lead to different phenotypes: classical Menkes disease or occipital horn syndrome.* Am J Hum Genet 2000;66(4) 1211-20.

[61]   Kennerson, M.L., et al. *Missense mutations in the copper transporter gene ATP7A cause X-linked distal hereditary motor neuropathy.* Am J Hum Genet 2010;86(3) 343-52.

[62]   Lepori, M.B., et al. *Mutation analysis of the ATP7B gene in a new group of Wilson's disease patients: contribution to diagnosis.* Mol Cell Probes 2012;26(4) 147-50.

[63]   Ferenci, P. *Regional distribution of mutations of the ATP7B gene in patients with Wilson disease: impact on genetic testing.* Hum Genet 2006;120(2) 151-9.

[64] Schushan, M., et al. *A structural model of the copper ATPase ATP7B to facilitate analysis of Wilson disease-causing mutations and studies of the transport mechanism.* Metallomics 2012;4(7) 669-78.

[65] Fatemi, N. and B. Sarkar. *Structural and functional insights of Wilson disease copper-transporting ATPase.* J Bioenerg Biomembr 2002;34(5) 339-49.

[66] Achila, D., et al. *Structure of human Wilson protein domains 5 and 6 and their interplay with domain 4 and the copper chaperone HAH1 in copper uptake.* Proc Natl Acad Sci U S A 2006;103(15) 5729-34.

[67] Banci, L., et al. *Solution structures of the actuator domain of ATP7A and ATP7B, the Menkes and Wilson disease proteins.* Biochemistry 2009;48(33) 7849-55.

[68] Banci, L., et al. *Metal binding domains 3 and 4 of the Wilson disease protein: solution structure and interaction with the copper(I) chaperone HAH1.* Biochemistry 2008;47(28) 7423-9.

[69] Dmitriev, O., et al. *Solution structure of the N-domain of Wilson disease protein: distinct nucleotide-binding environment and effects of disease mutations.* Proc Natl Acad Sci U S A 2006;103(14) 5302-7.

[70] Fatemi, N., et al. *NMR characterization of copper-binding domains 4-6 of ATP7B.* Biochemistry 2010;49(39) 8468-77.

[71] Gourdon, P., et al. *Crystal structure of a copper-transporting PIB-type ATPase.* Nature 2011;475(7354) 59-64.

[72] Gonzalez-Castejon, M., et al. *Functional non-synonymous polymorphisms prediction methods: current approaches and future developments.* Curr Med Chem 2011;18(33) 5095-103.

[73] Squitti, R., et al. *In silico investigation of the ATP7B gene: insights from functional prediction of non-synonymous substitution to protein structure.* Biometals 2014;27(1) 53-64.

[74] Squitti, R., et al. *Linkage disequilibrium and haplotype analysis of the ATP7B gene in Alzheimer's disease.* Rejuvenation Res 2013;16(1) 3-10.

[75] Squitti, R., et al. *ATP7B variants as modulators of copper dyshomeostasis in Alzheimer's disease.* Neuromolecular Med 2013;15(3) 515-22.

[76] Bucossi, S., et al. *Association of K832R and R952K SNPs of Wilson's Disease Gene with Alzheimer's Disease.* J Alzheimers Dis 2012;29(4) 913-9.

[77] Bucossi, S., et al. *Intronic rs2147363 variant in ATP7B transcription factor-binding site associated with Alzheimer's disease.* J Alzheimers Dis 2013;37(2) 453-9.

[78] Gupta, R.K., et al. *Transcriptional control of preadipocyte determination by Zfp423.* Nature 2010;464(7288) 619-23.

[79] Van Dyck, F., et al. *PLAG1, the prototype of the PLAG gene family: versatility in tumour development (review).* Int J Oncol 2007;30(4) 765-74.

[80] Squitti, R. and R. Polimanti. *Copper Hypo*thesis in the Missing Hereditability of Sporadic Alzheimer's Disease: ATP7B Gene as Potential Harbor of Rare Variants. J Alzheimers Dis 2012;29(3) 493-501.

Permissions

All chapters in this book were first published in AD, by InTech Open; hereby published with permission under the Creative Commons Attribution License or equivalent. Every chapter published in this book has been scrutinized by our experts. Their significance has been extensively debated. The topics covered herein carry significant findings which will fuel the growth of the discipline. They may even be implemented as practical applications or may be referred to as a beginning point for another development.

The contributors of this book come from diverse backgrounds, making this book a truly international effort. This book will bring forth new frontiers with its revolutionizing research information and detailed analysis of the nascent developments around the world.

We would like to thank all the contributing authors for lending their expertise to make the book truly unique. They have played a crucial role in the development of this book. Without their invaluable contributions this book wouldn't have been possible. They have made vital efforts to compile up to date information on the varied aspects of this subject to make this book a valuable addition to the collection of many professionals and students.

This book was conceptualized with the vision of imparting up-to-date information and advanced data in this field. To ensure the same, a matchless editorial board was set up. Every individual on the board went through rigorous rounds of assessment to prove their worth. After which they invested a large part of their time researching and compiling the most relevant data for our readers.

The editorial board has been involved in producing this book since its inception. They have spent rigorous hours researching and exploring the diverse topics which have resulted in the successful publishing of this book. They have passed on their knowledge of decades through this book. To expedite this challenging task, the publisher supported the team at every step. A small team of assistant editors was also appointed to further simplify the editing procedure and attain best results for the readers.

Apart from the editorial board, the designing team has also invested a significant amount of their time in understanding the subject and creating the most relevant covers. They scrutinized every image to scout for the most suitable representation of the subject and create an appropriate cover for the book.

The publishing team has been an ardent support to the editorial, designing and production team. Their endless efforts to recruit the best for this project, has resulted in the accomplishment of this book. They are a veteran in the field of academics and their pool of knowledge is as vast as their experience in printing. Their expertise and guidance has proved useful at every step. Their uncompromising quality standards have made this book an exceptional effort. Their encouragement from time to time has been an inspiration for everyone.

The publisher and the editorial board hope that this book will prove to be a valuable piece of knowledge for researchers, students, practitioners and scholars across the globe.

List of Contributors

Rita Moretti
Clinica Neurologica, Responsabile Ambulatorio Complicanze Internistiche Cerebrali, Dipartimento Universitario Clinico di Scienze Mediche, Chirurgiche e della Salute, Università degli Studi di Trieste, Italy

Arianna Sartori and Beatrice Baso
Clinica Neurologica, Dipartimento Universitario Clinico di Scienze Mediche, Chirurgiche e della Salute, Università degli Studi di Trieste, Italy

Silvia Gazzin
Area Science Park, FIF, Basovizza, Ospedale di Cattinara, Trieste, Italy

Wim Waterink
Faculty of Psychology and Educational Sciences, Open University of the Netherlands, The Netherlands

Susan van Hooren
Faculty of Psychology and Educational Sciences, Open University of the Netherlands, The Netherlands
Zuyd University of Applied Sciences, Heerlen, The Netherlands

José C. Fernández-Checa
Department of Cell Death and Proliferation, Instituto Investigaciones Biomedicas de Barcelona, CSIC, Barcelona, and Liver Unit-Hospital Clinic-IDIBAPS, Spain
Centro de Investigación Biomédica en Red (CIBERehd), Barcelona, Spain
University of Southern California Research Center for Alcohol Liver and Pancreatic Diseases and Cirrhosis, Keck School of Medicine, USC, Los Angeles, CA, USA

Genaro Gabriel Ortiz, Erika D. González-Renovato, Angélica Sánchez-López, Dhea G. Nuño-Penilla and Juan P. Sánchez-Luna
División de Neurociencias. Centro de Investigación Biomédica de Occidente (CIBO), Instituto Mexicano del Seguro Social (IMSS). Guadalajara, Jalisco, México

Fermín P. Pacheco-Moisés
Departamento de Química, Centro Universitario de Ciencias Exactas e Ingenierías. Universidad de Guadalajara. Guadalajara, Jalisco, México

Luis Figuera
División de Genética. Centro de Investigación Biomédica de Occidente, Instituto Mexicano del Seguro Social. Guadalajara, Jalisco, México

Miguel A. Macías-Islas, L. Javier Flores-Alvarado, Irma E. Velázquez- Brizuela and Alfredo Célis de la Rosa
Centro Universitario de Ciencias de la Salud. Universidad de Guadalajara. Guadalajara, Guadalajara, Jalisco, México

Mario Mireles-Ramírez
Departamento de Neurología. Unidad Médica de Alta Especialidad (UMAE)- Hospital de Especialidades; Centro Médico Nacional de Occidente. Instituto Mexicano del Seguro Social (IMSS). Guadalajara, Jalisco, México

Jiannan Wu, Yi Wang, Ping Li, Nannan Wei, Zhiquan Zhao and Huimin Liang
Laboratory of Brain Function and Molecular Neurodegeneration, Institute for Brain Science Research, School of Life Sciences, Henan University, Kaifeng, China

Zhenzhen Liu and Jianshe Wei
Laboratory of Brain Function and Molecular Neurodegeneration, Institute for Brain Science Research, School of Life Sciences, Henan University, Kaifeng, China
Institute of Neuroscience, Henan Polytechnic University, Jiaozuo, China

Xinxin Hou, Qingling Zhang and Peifu Li
Institute of Neuroscience, Henan Polytechnic University, Jiaozuo, China

Amany Mohamed, Kevan Smith and Elena Posse de Chaves
Department of Pharmacology, University of Alberta, Edmonton, AB, Canada
Neuroscience and Mental Health Institute, University of Alberta, Edmonton, AB, Canada

Carlo Salustri
Institute of Cognitive Sciences and Technologies (CNR), Fatebenefratelli Hospital, Isola Tiberina, Rome, Italy

Mariacristina Siotto
Don Carlo Gnocchi Foundation ONLUS, Milan, Italy

Serena Bucossi
Laboratory of Neurodegeneration, IRCCS San Raffaele
Pisana, Rome, Italy

Rosanna Squitti
Laboratory of Neurodegeneration, IRCCS San Raffaele
Pisana, Rome, Italy
Fatebenefratelli   Foundation,   AFaR   Division;
Fatebenefratelli Hospital, Isola Tiberina, Rome, Italy

Index

Q
Quetiapine Dosage, 7

S
Senile Plaques, 39, 61-63, 68, 70, 78, 140
Sexual Behaviour, 15-20, 22-23
Subcortical Vascular Dementia, 1-2
Synaptic Transmission, 101-102, 128

T
Tau Protein, 24, 51, 62-63, 72, 78-83, 85-87, 89, 91, 93, 95, 141

Trehalose, 85, 95-96

U
Ubiquinone, 92, 99, 114, 119, 140, 143

V
Vascular Dementia, 1-3, 9, 12, 14, 17, 65
Vasculitis, 3

Z
Zaragozic Acid, 106

www.ingramcontent.com/pod-product-compliance
Lightning Source LLC
Chambersburg PA
CBHW050459200326
41458CB00014B/5232